'Play Can Help' Series

FUN WITHOUT FATIGUE

Books by the same author

In this series

Look at it This Way   ISBN 0 7506 3895 8
Fingers and Thumbs   ISBN 0 7506 2524 4

Also

Play Helps (Fourth Edition)   ISBN 0 7506 2522 8

Commissioning editor: Heidi Allen
Desk editor: Claire Hutchins
Production controller: Chris Jarvis
Development editor: Robert Edwards
Cover designer: Alan Studholme

'Play Can Help' Series

FUN WITHOUT FATIGUE

Toys and Activities for Children
with Restricted Movement and Limited Energy

Roma Lear

Illustrated by Jill Hunter
and
Rebecca Finn

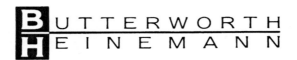

BUTTERWORTH
HEINEMANN

OXFORD AUCKLAND BOSTON JOHANNESBURG MELBOURNE NEW DELHI

Butterworth-Heinemann
Linacre House, Jordan Hill, Oxford OX2 8DP
225 Wildwood Avenue, Woburn, MA 01801-2041
A division of Reed Educational and Professional Publishing Ltd

℟ A member of the Reed Elsevier plc group

First published 2001

© Roma Lear 2001

British Library Cataloguing in Publication Data
A catalogue record for this book is available from the British Library

ISBN 0 7506 2525 2

For information on all Butterworth-Heinemann publications visit our website at www.bh.com

Transferred to digital printing in 2006.

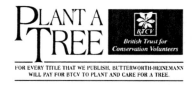

PLANT A TREE

FOR EVERY TITLE THAT WE PUBLISH, BUTTERWORTH-HEINEMANN
WILL PAY FOR BTCV TO PLANT AND CARE FOR A TREE.

Contents

Acknowledgements

My grateful thanks to Jill Norris who, in the late 1960s, started the first toy library in the UK for children with special needs and founded our present National Association of Toy and Leisure Libraries.

I am also indebted to:

- All the children who, over the years, have unwittingly supplied the material for this book.
- All the therapists and parents who have shared their ideas with me for the benefit of other children. You will find their names scattered throughout the book. The royalties earned from their contributions will benefit the National Association of Toy and Leisure Libraries.
- All my toy library friends and the staff at NATLL for their encouragement, suggestions and advice.
- Jill Hunter for her delightful illustrations, and Stuart Wynn-Jones, Anita Jackson and Caroline Gould for supplementary pictures, many of which have already appeared in my previous books. Additional delights to this book are the ten new illustrations by Rebecca Finn.
- Ann Kirk for her good-humoured and meticulous editing.
- And particularly to my husband, John, who has acted as critic and sounding board throughout the writing of this book.

Disclaimer

Every effort has been made to ensure that the information in this book is accurate, informed and as up-to-date as possible at the time of going to press. The author and publisher can neither be held liable for any errors or omissions, nor for any consequences of using inappropriately the toys and activities suggested.

Introduction to the 'Play Can Help' series

This series of three books is based on 'Play Helps, Fourth Edition'. That book is a collection of toys and activities which are relevant to children with a variety of play needs. In the 'Play Can Help' series, those ideas relating to a specific disability have been grouped together in one (cheaper!) book, and many more items are new to the present book. The first volume, 'Look at it This Way' was concerned with play for children with a visual impairment. The second, 'Fingers and Thumbs' gave ideas for toys and activities for those with a hand-function problem. Now comes the third book, 'Fun Without Fatigue'. This one is written for children who have, for whatever reason, restricted movement and limited energy. Every Paediatric Occupational Therapist and Hospital Play Specialist will be able to think of children who fall into one or both of these categories, sometimes for the whole of their childhood and, sometimes, while convalescing from a serious operation or illness.

My attention was first drawn to the special needs of this group of children when, many years ago, a little boy of three joined the toy library at Kingston-upon-Thames. He had brittle bones. His mother searched the cupboards for suitable toys, but at that time all were too large or too strong and heavy for him to manage. For this child, even Dinky toys were not suitable, because of their weight. Fortunately, I had tucked away a collection of celluloid farm animals. In those far off days, toys made from this flammable substance had not been banned. The animals formed the basis of a farm. With a little ingenuity, his mother and I soon concocted some farm buildings from cardboard boxes and made little fields from pieces of fabric. (Brown corduroy makes a convincing ploughed field and green terry towelling a realistic meadow! A tea packet made a splendid stable for the horse!) Each time the little boy visited the toy library, I tried to have an addition to the farm ready for him. It is amazing how many different ways a piece of paper can be folded! Later I attained a City and Guilds Certificate in toy making and during the last two years of the four-year course I was able to experiment with toys for 'frail' children. The basic requirements for such toys were, I felt, small size—so that they could be played with in a confined space, light weight—so that they did not require too much physical effort and, of course, they must be interesting and fun to play with. Many of my experiments were tried out on various children, mostly members of the Kingston-upon-Thames Toy Library for children with special needs, and the patients of my Paediatric Occupational Therapist friends. The best ideas have ended up in 'Fun Without Fatigue'.

This book is an attempt to increase the possible play activities for children for whom robust physical play is not an option. Some may have learning difficulties, others may one day qualify for Brain of Britain. I hope I have covered as many eventualities as possible in my attempt to combat the boredom that children with physical restrictions often suffer.

August 2001   Roma Lear

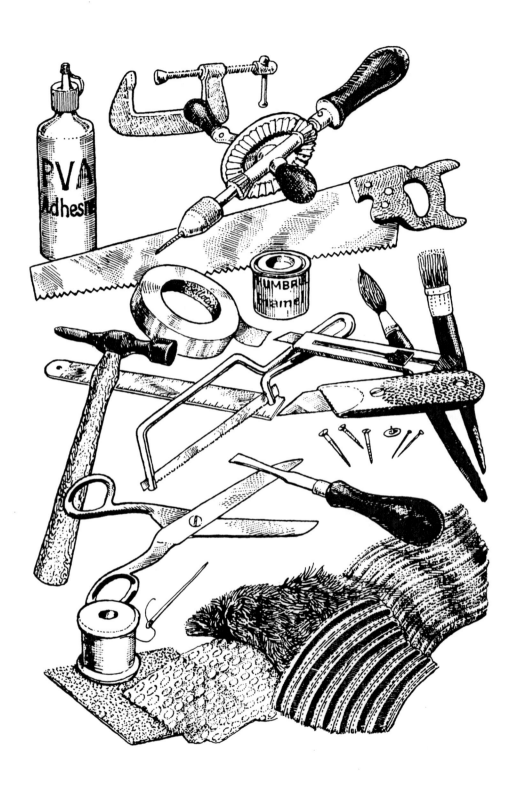

Before you begin

I hope you will find many toys in this book that will be both fun to make and, to play with. I have spent many years creating toys for children with special needs and, while fun has been the first consideration, I have also listened to my professional friends, and tried to help them sugar a therapeutic pill or two through play. I guess many of the children who handle the toys described in this book will do so gently and carefully. This may not be the case with their friends or siblings! SAFETY FIRST must always be the paramount concerns of any toy maker.

The great advantage in *making* toys—apart from the fun of it—is that each one is unique and can be tailor-made to suit the needs of the child. For one with limited movement and energy, size and weight are, of course, important considerations. You may need to scale down my suggested measurements or, perhaps, use alternative materials—like paper instead of card, if you think that would work as well.

The toys have been classified as *Instant*, *Quick* or *Long-lasting*. The *Instant* category is self-explanatory—think of the saucepan and wooden spoon 'drum' so beloved by busy toddlers. *Quick* toys should be made in an evening or less and, of course, *Long-lasting* include the potential family heirloom toys that can take as long as you like!

If you are new to toymaking, here are a few tips which may help you achieve really satisfactory results.

- Always use the best materials you can find. Choose birch plywood or MDF (Medium Density Fibreboard) for wooden toys. Both sand down well—no splinters or rough edges.
- Use new fabric. It is stronger than some which has been through the washing machine many times. If you think it necessary, use it double or back it with calico for extra strength.
- Pay attention to seams. Stitch them twice and oversew (or zig-zag) the edges to prevent the seams from splitting. Always fasten off very securely.
- Use button thread to attach all buttons.
- PVA adhesive is excellent for sticking paper and card. Some toys need a stronger adhesive and I have suggested a suitable one in the Materials section under the toy in question where I think it must be used.
- All paints and felt pens bearing the CE mark and sold as suitable for school use will be non-toxic. Humbrol enamel, sold in small tins for painting models etc., comes in bright colours, dries quickly and is safe to use on toys.
- Polyurethane varnish is non-toxic when dry. Two or three coats will form a hard, protective covering and make the toy wipeable—possibly even washable.
- Polyester fibre for soft toys is sold at craft shops etc. The bag should be marked 'Suitable for toy making' and bear the CE safety mark.

All that remains is for me to wish you well with your toymaking. You may go for a five minute wonder (like the paper helicopter—great fun while it lasts, but will soon end up in the bin,) or you may choose a more durable toy (like the peg bus), which may give pleasure to many children over the years. I believe there is room in the day for both. Obviously circumstances alter cases and the choice is yours!

Making play possible

KEEPING TOYS WITHIN REACH

Everyone caring for children with special needs is likely to have discovered how difficult it can be to keep toys within the reach of the child who is playing with them—and, occasionally, out of reach of the child who shouldn't be! The children for whom this book is intended are sure to need this kind of help at some time or another. Perhaps their toys may need suspending within easy reach, or keeping within a restricted space. They may even need some simple adaptations, like the application of a strip of magnetic tape perhaps. In this chapter you will find some ideas which have proved helpful to children with limited mobility and restricted reach. Perhaps one of them may be just the thing to solve you child's play problem too.

Some ways of suspending toys

An Elastic Luggage Strap

Instant

This useful and unusual toy-holder has strong hooks at both ends and can be stretched across a cot. It is easy to remove when the cot side needs lowering. It should be under slight tension to prevent sagging, so it is wise to measure between the rails before buying. Hang some toys with tape or string, but use elastic for others so that, when these are pulled and released, they will bob about.

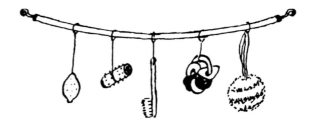

An Elastic Washing Line

Instant

Jeanette Maybanks

Here is an easy but effective way of suspending toys at any height. The brainwave came from a busy Mum who wanted to amuse her baby while he was still at the precrawling stage and floorbound on a rug. The idea could be used for any child who needs to play in a similar position. Just hang

4

a length of elastic between two suitable points—the rungs of chairs might do. At intervals along it, attach strong bulldog clips (from large stationers or office equipment suppliers). As the name suggests, these clips grip very firmly and will withstand a fair amount of tugging. From the clips, dangle anything suitable! Perhaps a handkerchief, a brilliantly coloured sock with a rattle in the toe, a soft toy on some ribbon or a glove with a little bell in one of the fingers.

A Plastic Garden Chain

Instant and long-lasting

Here is another way of stringing toys in a row, either for a child in a cot or for one lying on the floor. The chain is sold at every garden centre. It looks attractive and, of course, is very strong—and washable! When it is fixed firmly in position, simply tie toys to the links, position the child comfortably and let her have a go.

Goal Posts

Long-lasting

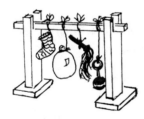

This idea is borrowed from the football pitch. A child can lie between the posts and easily reach all the delights that hang from the crossbar. The posts are slotted into sturdy feet (or fixed with brackets) so that the whole frame is very stable. The crossbar fits into grooves at the top of the posts and, at the end of playtime, the whole contraption can be taken apart for easy storage.

The Whirly Line

Instant

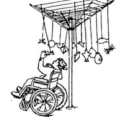

When the warm weather is here and the washing is out of the way, why not use the whirly line as an outdoor toy-holder? The fact that it revolves adds to its attraction. A determined child can tug his way to the toy of his choice.

Suggestions for Bits and Bobs to Hang

Instant

Select as appropriate:

- A balloon. Sausage-shaped ones are easier to hit. To minimise the risk of the balloon popping, do not over-inflate. A few grains of rice inside, or a small bell, will make it even more exciting.

- A bunch of ribbons or bright, non-fray strips of material.
- Any plastic bottle with a handle and something (safe) inside to rattle. Fix the lid on with a dab of plastic glue, e.g. U-Hu.
- A sock with something tactile in the toe, such as a rattle, a fir cone, or a squeaky toy. Stitch across the top of the sock.
- A string of large buttons, perhaps with a bell (from the pet shop) added here and there.
- A plastic sweet jar containing something interesting, such as coloured cotton reels, ping-pong balls or cat balls with a bell inside.
- An 'octopus' made from four pairs of coloured tights stuffed with newspaper and tied together at the top.
- See if a plastic baby mirror appeals. This is large and shiny and has convenient holes round the edge from which to hang it.
- Hang up a *bunch* of rattles—much easier to biff or grab than a single one.
- Thread coloured cotton reels on a string. Join the ends together to form a loop.
- Use the lid from a Golden Syrup tin and punch a small hole near the rim. This lid is chosen because it is strong and shiny and has a well-turned edge. To make its rotations more noticeable, stick a circle of brightly-coloured Fablon or some stickers to one side.
- Make a tassel from a few lengths of string. Thread one or two large buttons on each string. Tie a knot below each button and leave a space before threading on the next one. When a child pulls a string or swipes the lot, the buttons should click together.
- Hang up an empty bag from a wine box, inflate it, and perhaps decorate it with stickers or strips of plastic (electrician's) tape.
- Look around the kitchen for likely objects. Even a wooden spoon could be a winner.

Suggested by Christine Cousins, Judy Denziloe, Margaret Gilmore, Alison Harland, Lilli Nielson, Fiona Priest, RNIB Advisors.

Keeping toys to hand

Instant

Pam Courtney,
Teacher

A child with more than one disability is likely to have difficulty in keeping his toys within reach. His movements may be limited or difficult to control. Like the children in Pam's care, he may have learning difficulties, perhaps combined with poor sight or hearing. It is not surprising that such a child may soon lose interest in his play. If he pushes his toys away with an involuntary movement, there they can stay—out of reach, out of sight and probably out of mind. He will be left with nothing to do until someone notices his plight. Pam has suggested two simple ways of overcoming this problem:

1. Playing on a Sloping Surface

If the child is playing on the floor and lying on one side, a sheet of hardboard can be placed between him and the wall. The far edge of the hardboard, next to the wall, is raised (prop it up on a telephone directory?) Now when toys are pushed away, they will slide back down to him.

2. Playing in a Baby Bath

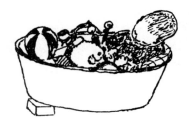

A small child who is able to sit up may find a baby bath makes a perfect 'child and toy container'. The high sides of the bath also help to keep toys to hand. Pam has found that for some children it is better to put plenty of toys in the bath—not just one or two. This bonanza cannot be ignored and should tempt the child to investigate and play. A plastic laundry basket could make an alternative to the baby bath. The basket has the added advantage that toys can be tied across the top or to the sides—useful if the child might otherwise end up sitting on them.

A Play Cushion

Quick

Susan Harvey,
Ann Hales-Tooke

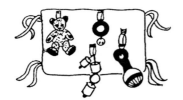

These pioneering Play Specialists made special cushions for their young patients who needed nursing in oxygen tents. In this situation the children continually lost their toys among the folds of the tent or dropped them on the floor. The play cushion evolved from an ordinary hospital pillow, already covered in washable plastic. This was given an attractive (and washable) cotton outer cover. Rings and loops were added to the front and tie-strings to the back. Now teethers, rattles and soft toys could be attached to the front for the child's delight, and the cushion kept safely in position by firmly attaching it to the cot bars, using the tie-strings at the back.

Method
- Use new material for the cover. It will be stronger.
- Make sure it is washable.
- Choose a plain colour. The toys will show up better.
- Do not over-clutter the play surface with rings and loops.
- Keep the strings that attach the toys to the pillow fairly short to avoid tangling.
- Remember to hold the child's interest by changing the toys as soon as they lose their appeal.

A Train Play Cushion

Long-lasting

Jean Gregg
Sarah Bondoux,
Play Specialists

As the illustration shows, this play cushion is made

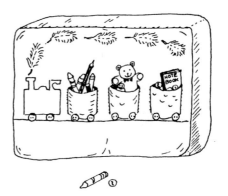

for older children and acts as a toy-holder. The removable cover is a restful blue and the little train that chugs across the front can contain small toys, crayons etc. It is firm and will stand alone. Its rigidity comes from the block of plastic foam inside, which measures approximately $60 \times 40 \times 8$ cm ($24 \times 16 \times 3$"). It can either be propped up between the child and the cot side (or the bed and the locker,) or it can be free-standing for a child lying on the floor.

A Play Table for Bed or Floor

Quick

Alison Wisbeach,
Occupational Therapist

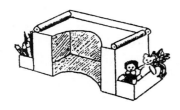

Children in hospital have tables that fit neatly over their beds. For the child who is nursed at home, Alison has thought up a quickly-made substitute— with the added advantage of storage space attached. She begins with a sturdy cardboard carton, (such as one from the Off Licence). She removes the top and turns it on its side, with the open end facing where the child will sit. As the picture shows, she cuts a crescent shape from the top and bottom of the box so that it will fit snugly round the child's body, and glues plastic pipe wrap to the three straight sides on the top of the box. This makes a retaining wall to prevent toys from falling off. Finally, she glues a shoe box to each side of the carton. These are to hold toys, books, art materials or what you will. Thus equipped, the child should have everything to hand for a happy play time.

A Play Corner

Quick

Judy Denziloe,
Director,
Action for Leisure

This is another simple way of keeping toys within reach. A carton from the supermarket is all you need. Remove the top and cut it in half diagonally—and there you are! It is possible you may care to add a few refinements like covering the box to make it look more attractive, or adding tapes so it can be anchored firmly to a table. Alternatively, place it in the corner of the room, so that the walls stop it from being pushed away or wedge it in place with a brick wrapped in cloth, or even use the telephone directory.

9

A Play Box

Quick

You will see from the illustration that this idea is similar to the one above. The outside of the box is covered with easily distinguishable textures, and there are rings on the inside for attaching toys. It is particularly useful for children with poor sight, but others can take to it for its novelty value.

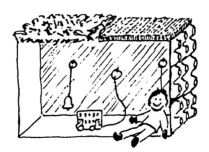

A Revolving Play Table

Instant and long-lasting

Imagine Mandy, a lively three-year-old, sitting in her custom-made wheelchair with its play tray in position in front of her. Because of her disability she had unusually short arms, and was only able to reach as far as the centre of the tray. Toys that strayed beyond the middle were out of reach. Tough!

A simple solution was to supply her with a cake icing turntable from the kitchen department of a High Street shop. By rotating the turntable, she instantly enlarged her play area and could reach any part she wanted. The turntable could also be placed to one side of the wheelchair. Now it could be used to hold the pieces of a puzzle, items of dolls' house furniture or whatever was top favourite at the moment.

If you have ever used a turntable while playing Scrabble, you will soon see other uses for this simple device. Obviously, it can come in handy when playing board games like Ludo or Snakes and Ladders. To meet a specific need, the surface of the turntable might be enlarged by covering it with a bigger circle of thick card or plywood, or by a square-shaped top. It could even have a lip added to stop small items from falling off.

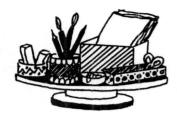

For older children with limited reach, the same idea can be used to provide storage space for pencils, felt pens, rubbers, rulers, glue, scissors, paper clips or what you will. Simply cover the surface of the turntable with containers of different sizes and shapes and, with a flick of the wrist, the child can bring the contents of them all to hand. Karen Paget, a Play Specialist in a busy Out-Patients Department, made one like this. She found it a boon for children sharing an activity table while waiting their turn for treatment.

A Reacher

Quick

Alison Wisbeach,
Occupational Therapist

Start with a length of dowel, drill a small hole in the top, and screw in a cup hook. You have made a simple 'reacher' which will soon pull straying toys back into play again. Of course, the thickness, length and weight of the dowel can be chosen with the requirements of the child in mind.

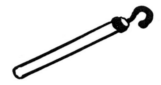

A Play Pinny

Quick

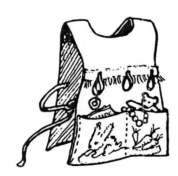

Here is another toy-holder, which really comes into its own if a child has to make a long journey. When he is strapped in a car seat, keeping him amused as the miles pass by can be quite a problem. The pinny is particularly useful for a small child, but it can also be appreciated by an older one—even if he has the advantage of a play tray attached to his car seat (corner smartly and toys can scatter!).

As the picture shows, the basic pattern is just an oblong of material with a hole for the child's head cut in it. Have the material about as wide as the child's shoulders. Before you cut out the head hole, either turn up one end to make the pockets or, if the fabric is not reversible, cut off a strip and add it to the front. Make a row of stitching down the centre, so that there is a pocket for each hand. Turn

11

in the side and bottom back seams. Cut out head hole and bind it. Try it for size! If it is too large, the pinny will slip off the child's shoulders; if too small, it will be a struggle to get it on and he will surely protest! Add some loops of tape to the front for attaching toys—not more than three or they may tangle together. It is a good idea to sew a reinforcing strip behind these loops, for they may have to withstand a fair amount of tugging. Add tie-strings to the sides. These stop the pinny from rucking up. Further treasures can be stored in the pockets.

SOME LIFESAVERS

If the above ways of making play possible are not suitable or appealing, here are a few 'Lifesavers'

- Give the child some means of signalling for help if desperately required. Perhaps the Ship's Bell on p. 30.
- Devise a way of organising toys so that they don't all get lost among the bedclothes (*see* Play Cushion above). Some parents use a peg bag as a toy-holder, others pin a carrier bag to the sheet. (The latter can be an excellent way of disposing of rubbish after a cutting-out session for example. Just drop the trimmings in the carrier bag.)
- A pencil on a string, tied to the bed head, may prevent a crisis.
- If a toy with many small pieces is top favourite, try putting a picture frame (without the glass, of course) on the table. It should keep everything like Lego bricks, or the tiny accessories for 'Play People' within bounds.

Begin at the beginning

Imagine you are cradling in your arms a tiny baby, only a few weeks old. The chances are you will be making eye contact and exchanging smiles. If this happens, you will know that the baby can now use his eyes to focus on a nearby object that attracts him—in this case your face. He may also be developing his sense of hearing, and will appreciate the soothing, crooning sounds, which you are probably making.

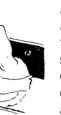

Assuming our baby is now able to use both his eyes and his ears, through them he will start to learn about the world around him. Some children may be at this stage for much longer than others, and over time may need a large assortment of sights and sounds presented to them. This chapter is concerned with looking and listening. It contains a collection of ideas suitable for copying, or for adapting to individual needs.

LEARNING TO LOOK

Through our eyes we acquire much of the information we need for living skills, learning and pleasure. The tiny baby who has learnt to focus on and recognise his Mother's face has passed a major milestone in his development. From then on, he will start to recognise and build up a memory bank of observations. I am reminded of Rachel, a little girl lying on her plaster shell in the Orthopaedic Hospital where I then worked. At that time, her vision was restricted by the walls of the ward and what she could see from her prone position but, one afternoon, I discovered she had a wealth of memories in her mind's eye. Given a tray and a new pack of Plasticine, she spent a happy couple of hours recreating a seaside scene. Mum sat on a rug reading, with the picnic beside her. Dad, trousers rolled up and knotted handkerchief on his head, paddled in the shallows, while the baby, navigating between sand castles and their busy creators, crawled over the sand towards him. The scene was full of life and interest. This little girl had certainly learnt to look.

MOBILES

Perhaps little cave babies, lying on their sabre-toothed tiger rugs at the beginning of history, gurgled happily as they watched fluffy white clouds drift across the mouth of the cave and leaves flutter in the breeze. Unless someone has thoughtfully provided him with a mobile, the modern baby lying in his cot, may only have the boring white ceiling to stare at. This situation can be part of the daily lives of older children too. Perhaps they are unable to move independently. They may be sick, or injured and temporarily in plaster. They must stay where they are put. Under such circumstances a colourful mobile can soothe, intrigue and certainly help to relieve tedium. Adults like mobiles too! Just because a child has outgrown the one she had as a baby, it does not mean that this delightful form of decoration must no longer be part of the décor. There are mobiles of every description in the shops—at a price. Delightful as these may be, they can have their limitations, for they may be too small or too complicated for a child to see easily. A single bold and gaudy shape may be more to her taste. 'Variety is the spice of life' as the saying goes, and this certainly applies to mobiles. They should never be regarded as a permanent fixture, but be changed, or perhaps used in rotation, as soon as they lose their child appeal. This could make a hole in the budget! How much more satisfactory to enlist the help of the family and indulge in a spot of creative Do It Yourself. Assuming this course of action appeals to you, and that you are new to mobile-making, here are a few tips before you begin.

Making a Mobile

Have a plan of action
This is always a wise move. A few decisions made in advance will avoid frustration. Assembling the materials you plan to use will ultimately save time, and help you to visualise the finished product. If time is scarce, don't be too ambitious. Before you begin, consider all the points that follow.

Decide on the subject
The mobile may be for an individual child or for a group. The likely viewing audience will determine its size and its theme.

Consider the practical points
1. *Where will you hang your mobile?* Obviously it must be at the right distance and height to be seen comfortably—for that is the whole purpose of the exercise. It is meant to move gently and so should be hung in a slight draught. A good position might be in line with the door, by a window or near the central heating.
2. *How will you hang it?* Commercial baby mobiles come fitted with a clamp to attach to the cot rail. If you have one of these, it may be possible to make use of it. In a room, a length of string can be stretched across one corner. Tie it to a couple of cup hooks screwed into the picture rail. For safety reasons never hang a mobile from a light fitting—tempting as that might be! In one children's hospital, brackets have been attached to the wall, out of reach of

the nurses' heads but within the line of vision of the child in bed. Only consider making a large and heavy mobile for a classroom or hospital ward if there is a ceiling hook or rafter available. You must be confident it can be suspended with complete safety.

3. *How will you display the shapes*? (The word 'shapes' here does not necessarily mean geometric ones. It refers to all the hanging bits and pieces.)

Here are some popular methods for small mobiles:

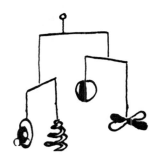

- *A coat-hanger*. Paint a wooden one white to smarten it up. Drill a few holes at intervals along it, or cut some notches in the top, to prevent the strings from bunching together or falling off. If you use a wire coat-hanger, keep the strings in place with Sellotape.
- *Two thin garden canes*. Cut them about 30 cm (12") long. Bind them together in the centre in the shape of a X. The mobile will hang from the centre of the X while the shapes dangle from the four corners and from the centre.
- *Wire*. If you want your mobile to hang in a cluster, as in the illustration, you will need short lengths of wire with the ends turned up.

  Start off with one 'bar'. From that one hang two more. These can either hold two shapes or perhaps one shape and another bar. The more ambitious you are, the more difficult it is to make the mobile balance—so allow time for assembly! If one end of a bar dips downwards, either shorten the string on the shape or adjust the position of the string that suspends the bar. This is like balancing a see-saw! You will find a very little adjustment will make all the difference.

Here are some suggestions for hanging large mobiles. Remember the safety factor!

- *A plastic hoop*. Tie three or four strings to the

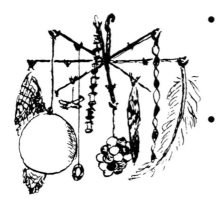

hoop. One should be longer than the others. Knot all the strings together and check that the hoop hangs level, then suspend it by the longer string. Tie the shapes to the rim.

- *A drip-dry carousel from a shop.* This comes complete with a hanging hook and pegs on the spokes for clipping on the shapes. It should have no balance problems but, if it tilts, try rearranging the shapes with the heavier ones nearer the centre.

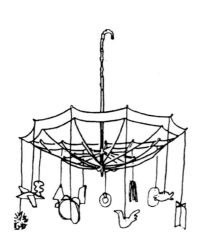

- *An old umbrella.* This makes an ideal mobile holder for a large area. Our Toy Library recently celebrated its twentieth birthday, and we made use of this method as part of the decorations. Our hall has convenient rafters so hanging them safely was not a problem. For several weeks beforehand, we collected jaded umbrellas with shabby covers or the odd bent spoke. With the children 'helping', we made large cardboard shapes of toys—dolls, teddies, trains, boats, balls, rattles ... you name it, we made it! The shapes were coloured both sides and strings attached. Then we prepared the umbrellas. The easiest way was to open them out, then cut away the bulk of the cover, leaving about 5 cm (2") round the edge to keep the spokes evenly spaced. (If you remove all the cover, the spokes will flop about and have to be repositioned at equal distances from each other. This can be a tiresome job.) The final task was to tie the shapes to the spokes, climb the ladder and fix our jolly brollies to the rafters.

Methods and Materials

Having disposed of most of the practical problems, now we come to the fun part of *making the shapes*. This is the time to be creative. Decide on the theme for your mobile. Avoid spherical or cylindrical shapes unless you need them for a specific purpose—to represent the sun perhaps? They will not rotate like flat ones.

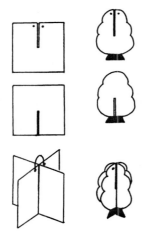

If you want to be a little more adventurous with a flat shape, try cutting it out twice. In one, cut a slot from the top to the middle, and in the other, from the bottom to the middle. Slot them together at right angles as in the diagram. Hang from the first shape (with the slot in the top half). If you hang from the second, the first will probably drop out.

Mobiles are usually made to be watched but not touched. If this is the case with yours, it is possible to use more unusual materials like feathers, sequins, painted egg shells, sweet wrappers or even fragile Christmas tree decorations—providing you are generous with the glue and there is no possibility of bits fluttering down on the child. If the mobile is likely to be handled, go for shapes made from card, wood or cloth.

What to hang on your mobile

If you are new to mobile making, you may appreciate a few ideas to start you off.

Cutting out a Single Large Shape and Decorating it

Quick

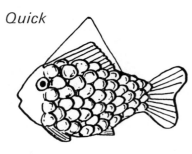

This is probably the easiest mobile of all and you can enlist the help of a child. Take a piece of cardboard and cut out a familiar shape such as a car, a house or a fish. Decorate both sides of the card appropriately.

Finding the suspension point of a large mobile can be a problem. No one wants to look at a house with subsidence or a car for ever going up hill! The solution is to hang the shape from a thread attached at two points, like a picture cord. Tie the suspending thread to this and the shape can be see-sawed like a picture on a nail, until it is hanging correctly.

Treasures from a Country Walk

Very quick

Imagine you have found a conker with its spiny shell, some acorns still attached to their cups, a feather and a cluster of fluffy old man's beard seeds. Tie them at intervals along a twig, hang it so that it balances—and you have a beautiful mobile to remind you of the walk. Of course, it will have a limited life, but this is a point in its favour. Its viewers will not have time to grow so bored with it that they stop looking!

A Flock of Birds

Quick

Bedelsford School

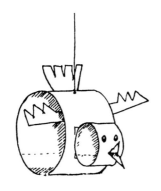

These attractive little birds hang in the corner of the room where the nursery children take their rest. They are made of white paper with only their orange beaks and black eyes to add a touch of colour. The effect is gentle and soothing—just right for rest time.

The body of each bird is made from a ring of paper (like a large napkin ring). The head is made from a smaller one. Stick these together. Make a beak from a diamond-shaped scrap of paper, colour it, fold it in half and stick it to the head. Mark in the eyes with black felt pen. If you want wings, cut them both out together and stick them to the inside of the body ring. (The birds at Bedelsford are wingless and look quite convincing!) Attach an upward-sweeping tail to give the bird a perky look—a drooping tail makes it look depressed!

A Shoal of Paper Fish

Quick

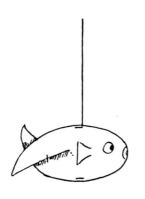

These fish have a chubby, three-dimensional look and are quite easy to make. Cut out two oval pieces of fairly stiff paper. Decorate them while they are still flat. You may like to make each side different—some fish are like that! One side could be dark blue and the other covered with diffraction paper. This would give a striking effect when the fish gently rotates on the end of its string.

In each fish shape cut a slit from the middle of the tail to roughly the middle of the body. Take the two parts of the tail and overlap them so that the points stick out beyond the body. Stick or staple them in place. The half body now bows out a little. If you want top or bottom fins, add them now, then staple or stick the two halves together. Hold them in place with a rubber band until the glue dries. If the fish tends to collapse on you at this stage, open it out and pad it with a little scrunched-up tissue paper. Add a dab of glue here and there to keep this in place. Attach the side fins. Finally, find the best position for the hanging thread. Poke a needle through the body in the place where you think it should go and see how it balances. Remember the fish do not all have to swim straight. The mobile looks more interesting if a few with independent spirits head for the surface of the water and others for the sandy bottom.

Another Shoal of (Felt) Fish

Fairly quick

It must be admitted that this mobile will take a little longer than the one above, but it is more robust. It makes a pretty present that can safely be sent through the post. The fish are made from scraps of different coloured felt and decorated with sequins. First make some paper patterns of fish shapes. If you need inspiration, look in fishy books or study the real thing at your local pet shop. Using the patterns, cut out each fish twice in felt. Sew on felt eyes and the sequins. It is easier to finish off properly at the back if you do this before the two halves are joined together—with stab stitch, over-sewing or buttonhole stitch. I like to incorporate the hanging thread as I stitch along the back of the fish. To make sure the thread will not pull out, I tie the bottom end to a tiny roll of felt and bury this in the body of the fish, making a few extra stitches either side of the thread for good measure. Before finishing off the stitching, insert a little polyester fibre to give the fish a chubbier shape.

A Mobile Within a Mobile

Quick

Susie Mason,
Toy Librarian

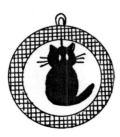

Susie knows a delightfully simple way of making a mobile where the centre shape moves independently from the outside. She starts with a round cheese box, and removes the centre, leaving the rim intact to make the frame. From the centre she cuts a shape—a face, flower, animal, boat, Christmas tree—or what you will. The shape is coloured both sides and hung in the centre of the frame which is also coloured both sides.

Mobiles with a Theme

A Weather Mobile
Here a yellow ping-pong ball might represent the sun. Clouds are easily cut from card and covered with fluffy cotton wool, or coloured grey for a rainy day. Strips of grey or black wool with glass beads on the end might represent raindrops, hung from a black cloud perhaps. A streak of lightning made from a zig-zag of card covered with diffraction paper looks impressive and flashes in the light. Snowflakes can be cut from a paper doily and stiffened with spray starch. A bunch of fine net gives an impression of fog.

A Birthday Mobile
This can be completed with the child's name, a cake, candles, presents and cards.

A Seasons Mobile
Make the shapes as appropriate. For winter you might choose a Christmas tree, a snowman, bare trees, robins or warm clothes like scarves and bobble hats. Let the children help to provide the inspiration.

A Festival Mobile
You are on your own here! There are so many festivals to celebrate, the choice is yours.

Some unusual mobiles

A Power-driven Mobile

Long-lasting

Have you ever poked a rubber band through both a cotton reel and a chunk of candle, anchoring it at both ends with a matchstick, wound it up and watched it crawl across the carpet? If so, you will understand the mechanism which keeps this mobile gently turning for a surprisingly long time.

You only need elementary carpentry skills, a fret saw, a drill and some sandpaper to make a power-driven mobile like the one illustrated.

Materials
- Scraps of plywood.
- Thin dowelling.
- A strong rubber band (dropped by the postman?)

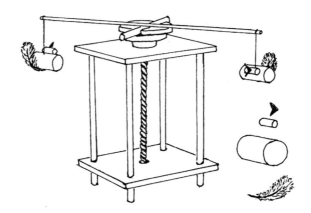

- A small piece of candle.
- A drinking straw.
- Paper and trimmings for the birds.
- A dab of glue and a scrap of Sellotape.

Method

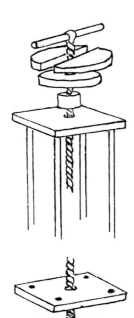

Cut two squares of plywood, say 10 cm × 10 cm (4"). Drill four holes in each corner of the base (to accommodate the dowel) and four in corresponding places partway through the top. Drill through the centre of each square to make the holes for the rubber band. Cut four equal lengths of dowel for the side supports. Allow for the feet and for the distance between the top and bottom squares, which should be about the same as the length of the elastic band. Cut two more short lengths of dowel. One will anchor the rubber band at the top. The other will act as a key to wind it up. The key needs to just fit between the supports or it will not turn easily. Cut two discs of plywood, say 7 cm (2½") diameter. Drill a hole in the centre of one and cut the other in half (*see* exploded illustration). Make a hole in the centre of the piece of candle. The easiest way of doing this without the risk of splitting it is to put a needle in a cork. Hold the cork, heat the needle and melt out a hole just large enough to take the rubber band.

Thread the rubber band up through the base and stop it from pulling through with the 'key' dowel. Then thread it up through the top square, the

23

candle and the bottom disc. Hold it there with the other short dowel. Glue the half circles to the bottom disc, each side of the dowel, with a gap between them. This makes it easier to replace the rubber band when it eventually snaps. Fix the straw across the top with Sellotape.

The Birds
These are made from two strips of paper as for the Bird Mobile on p. 20. Add a scrap of coloured feather (or paper) for the tails and hang one on each end of the drinking straw.

Turn the 'key' to twist the band. When it is crinkly, (and before it snaps!) wedge the key against one of the legs to stop it from unwinding. Stand back and enjoy the result. Children find this silent and gently rotating mobile riveting—and adults go for it in a big way!

Dancing Danglement

Quick

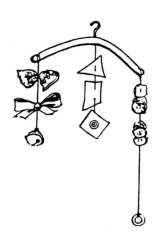

This is a mobile that does not rely on a draught to make it move. It is activated by 'baby power'. When the string is pulled, the mobile will bob about and set the noisemakers jangling.

Hang a coat-hanger out of reach of the child, but where he can see it easily. Tie on an assortment of noisy objects and some colourful ones. You might include a bunch of bells, a string of foil milk bottle tops, a rattle, a tassel of brightly-coloured ribbons, cellophane sweet wrappers tied in the middle to make them look like butterflies ... Make about three strings of these, with one considerably longer than the others. This is the one for the child to pull. Make it easy to grasp by tying a cotton reel or a large ring to the end. Make certain the strings cannot slip off the hanger. Either drill holes for them or cut notches in the top before you tie them on tightly.

A Bamboo Mobile

Long-lasting

This mobile can be used in two ways. In version one, it is hung out of reach, like the Dancing Danglement above, and the child pulls a string to make the noise. In version two (as shown on p. 25) it is hung within reach for a 'hands on' experience. The child runs his hands along the line of bamboo strips to make them strike together. The mobile is weather resistant (until the string rots), so it can be hung outside in the winter, from the branches of a bare tree near the window, where it could provide a welcome spot of colour on a dreary day.

If your time is limited, omit the scraping and painting stages and use the bamboo in its natural state. The mobile will not be so eye-catching, but the sound it makes will be equally attractive.

Materials

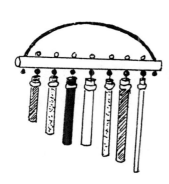

- A length of broomstick or thick dowelling for the support.
- Bamboo garden canes – say two.
- An old knitting needle.
- Paint. Acrylic is best, but poster will do.
- Polyurethane varnish.
- Thin nylon cord for suspending the support.
- Strong, thin thread for hanging the bamboo sections.
- Beads. Optional, but they make the bamboo sections hang better, and look pretty.

Method

Divide the bamboo canes into separate sections by cutting about 10 mm above each joint. The sections will be different lengths and thicknesses. This is good because they will all make a different sound. Discard any spoilt or faulty ones and keep about ten of the best. With a craft knife, scratch away the waxy surface on each section. (Work away from yourself and take care.) It is important to remove all the waxy surface or the paint will not stick properly, and will flake off when the sections knock together. Rub each section with sandpaper to make sure it is smooth and clean. Drill a small hole (just large enough to take the hanging thread) down through the joint at the top of each section. Remove any pith in the middle of the bamboo with a knitting needle. Hold the section up to your eye. You should now be able to see right through it. Poke the hanging thread through the hole in the joint and out through the bottom. Tie a VERY large knot on the end, or better still, thread it through a small bead and tie it on firmly. This will prevent the hanging thread from pulling out through the hole in the joint. Paint all the bamboo sections in bright colours and when they are dry protect them with at least two coats of Polyurethane varnish. Decide how you would like them to hang, and arrange them in a row. Leave a gap between each—about the width of a section—and measure the space they occupy. Cut the broomstick (or dowel) about 8 cm (3") longer. Drill holes at appropriate places along it, one for each section of bamboo and one at each end for the suspending cord. Tie each section to the hanger. If you use beads, thread one as a spacer between the section and the hanger and perhaps one on the top (as in the illustration). Finally, attach the suspending cord. Add the pull string if you are making version one.

A Compact Disc Mobile

Quick and long-lasting

Carole Sunter,
Teacher of Visually
Impaired Children,
Orkney

This unusual mobile is made from unwanted Compact Discs. It is not as noisy as the ones above, but visually it certainly has the 'Wow' factor! It catches the light beautifully and, if hung in sunlight, will reflect rainbow patterns on nearby walls. The fairly large surface area of each CD helps it to rotate and sway in the slightest air current. Should two bump together, the gentle noise they make is an added attraction.

Materials
- Old CDs, say six as in the picture.
- A small drill bit.
- Fishing line or strong thread.
- Brightly coloured paper or cloth for the backs of the CDs (if required).
- A curtain ring for the hanging loop.

Method
Choose one CD to be the spacer disc at the top of the mobile. Drill four equidistant holes near the circumference (use a small drill bit, or Carol says the disc may shatter.) Drill one small hole near the

circumference of each of the other five discs. Attach a fairly long hanging string to each one. You can cut off the surplus when the mobile is hanging as you want it. If the backs of the other discs are uninteresting, cover them with gaudy paper or cloth. Copydex or PVA adhesive will do this job.

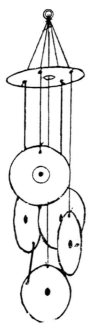

Assemble the mobile as illustrated—one disc on the longest string in the centre and the other four round the outside. The easiest way to do this is to tie a string to the curtain ring and let it dangle down. If no one is handy to hold it for you, rest a broomstick across the backs of two upright chairs and let the curtain ring hang from that. Thread the central disc (with the longest hanging thread) up through the spacer disc. Tie it to the curtain ring. At this stage, the spacer disc will flop over the central disc. Poke the hanging thread from one of the outer CDs up and through one of the holes in the spacer disc. Wind the thread over the edge and up through the hole again to prevent it slipping. Adjust the height of this outer disc so that it is hanging clear of the one in the centre. Tie the top of its string to the curtain ring. Repeat the process for the other three outer discs. Hang them at different levels for the best effect and freedom of movement. Ease the spacer disc up and nearer to the curtain ring. The weight of the four discs suspended round the edge will now keep it in position.

LOOKING LIFESAVERS

Even the most imaginative and dedicated teacher or carer can occasionally be at her wit's end for something simple and new to amuse her charge(s). For some children 'looking' is their main activity, and it is important to ring the changes. Scan your eye down the following list. Even if nothing on it is suitable for the child in question, it may start you thinking!

- Eye catching posters pasted on a ceiling. This was done to great effect at a school I once visited.

- Glow stars or shapes on the walls or ceiling may keep a wakeful child happy at night.
- When one of my own children was sick, I inadvertently left a bowl of water on the windowsill. We were both entranced by the Jack-a-dandies it reflected on the ceiling.
- Mirrors can come in handy for any child lying in awkward positions. A driving mirror fixed to the bed head or other strategic position and suitably angled might reflect who is coming through the door, or what is happening outside the window.
- On a wet day have races between the raindrops on the windowpane.
- Make shadows on the wall. All you need is a shaft of sunlight (or an anglepoise lamp), a little imagination, and some practice! Try something simple like a fluttering butterfly. Link your thumbs together for the body, keep your fingers straight and close together for the wings, get the angle right and off you go.
- A well-maintained fish tank is beautiful to look at, constantly changing and always interesting. One may be installed in your Dentist's waiting room for a very good reason. The gentle movement of the fish is both restful and makes for compulsive viewing.
- Watching things grow can give some children great pleasure, *see* 'Bringing the World to the Child' p. 107.
- Watching something move is always more fun than looking at a static object. Any toddler with a tin of bubble mixture and a bubble wand will soon demonstrate the truth of this! For a more permanent—and more easily seen 'bubble'—try a balloon, preferably tossed gently by an adult or hung where the movement of the air will make it sway gracefully.
- Table lamps with coloured oily shapes floating about inside the base are attractive as are fibre optic lights, disco balls and other delights found in the school sensory room.

Looking—with a friend

- Look intently at a picture, then hide it. Name as many items in it as possible. Have another look to check how many have been remembered.
- 'Torch Hee' is a splendid game for playing in bed in the dark. Each child has a torch. One child shines his beam on the wall and moves it about—not too fast. The other child tries to focus his beam on top of it. When successful, he shines his torch first and leads the next beam chase.

See also
Kim's Game, p. 98
A Convection Snake, p. 117
Pop-up dollies, pp. 119, 133
A Cup and Ball, p. 122

LEARNING TO LISTEN

Rattles

A rattle is often a baby's first real toy, and its origins are lost in the mists of time. I guess it has been around for as long as mankind—the first rattle was probably just a seed in a pod, or a bunch of bones tied together with a sinew! In its present colourful and hygienic shape, it is perfect for a first lesson in 'cause and effect'. Nothing will happen unless it is held firmly, turned this way and that, passed from hand to hand (dropped!) or simply waved about. Some children need this type of play for much longer than others. As a child grows bigger, and possibly stronger, baby rattles may no longer be exciting or appropriate. This is where a different sort of rattle can come in handy. Here are some suggestions.

A Rattle from an Orange Squash Bottle

Instant

(For a tiny child, a smaller mineral water bottle may be better.) This rattle is ideal for any child who has just learnt to sit up. Its size, light weight and transparency definitely give it child appeal. Its owner is

29

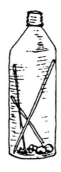

likely to spend ages just shaking it to make the loudest possible noise, and watching the contents bob about inside, then settle to the bottom.

Wash the bottle thoroughly. Before putting in the contents, make sure it is really dry. If any moisture remains inside, it may cause condensation. For safety reasons, it is best to insert edible items like spaghetti, lentils and rice. If you are certain the child will not manage to undo the lid, you might add a few coloured buttons, a small bell and balls of foil paper. These look attractive and can make a different noise. Once the contents are inside, squirt a little plastic adhesive—like U-Hu—inside the lid and screw it on firmly. This should deter all but the most inquisitive children from getting at the contents. Wait for the glue to dry before giving the rattle to its new owner.

A 'Ship's Bell' Rattle from an Inverted Treacle Tin

Quick

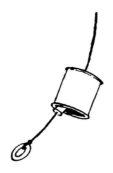

This rattle is capable of generating plenty of decibels! It can be either hand-held (by you) or tied to a cot play bar or—for a child lying on the floor—to the rung of a chair.

Materials
- A treacle tin.
- About 45 cm (18") string or piping cord. The latter looks more attractive and is pleasant to feel.
- A clapper. A wooden cotton reel is ideal—if you still have one! Failing that, use a macramé bead of about the same size, or a wooden brick with a hole drilled through it.

Method
Wash and dry the tin. (Keep the lid. It has a nicely turned lip and could come in handy for another toy!) Turn the tin upside down and punch a hole in the centre of the bottom. Thread the cord through the hole, keeping enough above the tin to hang it by. Tie a large knot for the tin to rest on. Without this, it will just slide off the string. Tie another knot outside the tin to keep it from sliding up the cord. Now thread on the clapper. It must be positioned so that it will

strike against the lip of the tin. Tie a knot in the cord, just below it to keep it in position. Tie a ring to the end of the cord to make it easier for the child to grasp. Perhaps make the tin look more attractive by giving it a coat of Humbrol enamel or covering it with a spare scrap of Fablon.

Some Small, Light Rattles

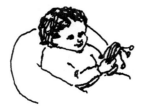

A tic-tac sweet container or similar
Put in a few grains of rice. Seal down the lid with plastic tape.

A dumb-bell rattle
This was made at the request of a therapist who needed a slender rattle for a baby born with one thumb tucked in. I used a short length of tube, (the width of the baby's palm) cut from an empty felt pen. I washed out the tube, then passed a length of round hat elastic down the centre and tied a bell to each end. I cut two circles from thin cotton fabric, gathered round the edge of each one, and stitched them over the bells like miniature mob caps. I covered the shaft of the rattle with a narrow strip of fabric, with the edges turned in. This strip also covered the edges of the circles and made a neat finish to this tiny rattle.

An empty film carton
This can soon be transformed into a small, light cylindrical rattle. A parent who attends our toy library showed me one she had made for her little daughter. Her carton contained a bell. Some holes were punched in the plastic (to let out the sound), and the lid replaced. Then the carton was encased in a crochet cover. This made it visually attractive, easier to hold and made sure the lid could not be removed.

An unusual twirly rattle
Invented by Alison Wisbeach, this rattle has been highly acclaimed by all the children who have received one! Its skeleton is a small metal egg

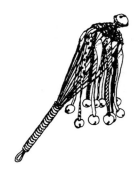

whisk. Short lengths of colourful ribbon, each with a bell sewn to one end, are stitched to alternate loops of wire. When the whisk is twirled, the ribbons fly out like the chairs on a fairground chair-a-plane. To ensure this happens, the ribbons must be prevented from crowding together at the end of the whisk. This can be done by backstitching in wool, over each loop of wire in turn, so forming a web which blocks in the end of the whisk. Press the web strands together and keep them in place with a few stitches between the loops of wire.

A Sound Matching Game

Long-lasting

This simple game is based on the film carton rattle above. These plastic containers with well-fitting lids (all with an identical and gaudy crochet cover) are an ideal size for small hands. The game is to have lots of them with various fillings inside. The children shake them in turn and discover which ones sound the same.

Materials
- Film cartons – say twelve, or as many as you need for your game.
- Noisy contents. Try rice, fish grit, milk bottle tops, a wooden bead, two buttons, bells, shells ... experiment with what you have to hand. Punch a few holes in each carton to help let out the sound.
- A ball of brightly-coloured wool.
- A suitably small crochet hook. The cover needs to fit tightly, so the stitches must be close together. (All the covers must be the same colour or the children are likely to sort them by sight and not by sound.)

Method
For young children, have say four cartons containing rice, four with fish grit (for a louder sound) and three empty. The children will probably try their hardest to make these rattle! It is interesting for them to experience silence.

For a more difficult game, arrange the cartons in pairs. Fill each pair as you choose, trying to keep the sounds as distinctive as possible. Rice or peas once inside the carton can sound remarkably alike. Replace the lids and crochet the covers. I work a circle the same size as the base, then carry on, without increasing, for the height of the carton. (The shape is rather like a miniature dustbin!) A separate crochet circle covers the top and is stitched firmly to the rest of the work. The carton is now safely encased in its woolly cover.

A Rattle Snake

Long-lasting

Like the real thing, this noisy reptile can be heard as well as seen. Its head and tail are filled with soft padding—in case the child waves it about and inadvertently hits himself! Various noisemakers are distributed along its body. If these are interspersed with interesting tactile sections, it makes for an even more attractive toy. The snake illustrated also has unfilled stripes between each section. This makes the snake suitably floppy and sinuous.

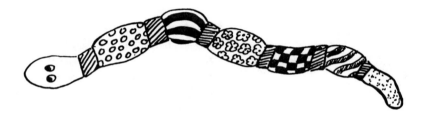

Materials
- Small pieces of strong, colourful and possibly textured material (e.g. fur fabric, corduroy or velvet) for the skin.
- A little polyester fibre to stuff the head and tail.
- Some noisemakers. Perhaps a film carton with a little fish grit inside, some bells or a cat ball (from the pet shop) a squeaker (from a craft shop) or even an unwanted small commercial rattle.
- Some tactile objects. Large buttons, bubbly plastic or an empty potato crisp bag, large beads, etc.
- Small scraps of black and white felt for the eyes.

33

Method

How long is the snake? As long as a piece of string! When making for an individual child, I think of a suitable length and weight for her to manage. If there are no specific requirements, the size can depend on the materials and time at my disposal.

First lay out the noisemakers and tactile objects which make up the 'innards' in the order in which you will use them—smaller ones nearer the tail. Then arrange the fabrics for the skin. Cut out the head. This is shaped like the toe of a sock. The body sections will vary in length according to their contents, and will look more snake-like if they gradually get narrower nearer the tail. All the 'innards' have to be inserted through the tail so this must be wide enough to accept the largest item. Start with the head. (Possibly add a hinge strip between each section as in the illustration.) Pin each section to the next, making sure it will be the right size to accept its 'innards', which will be inserted through the rounded tail end. Stitch the sections together. With the strip of fabric inside out, pin the snake together down the side, making sure the edges of the sections are in line. Before you sew up this side seam, try the snake skin for size and make sure the 'innards' will fit inside. Sew round the head and join up the side seam, leaving the end of the tail open. Turn the snake the right side out. Stuff the head with polyester fibre. Stitch across the body to keep this in place. If you have made a hinge, stitch across this too. Fill the first section with its 'innards' and stitch across as before. Continue like this all down the snake until you come to the tail. Stuff this with polyester fibre and finish off by hand. Add felt eyes.

A Home-made Telephone

Quick

For this you need a pair of treacle tins (or similar—with a turned and safe lip) and a fairly long piece of string. Punch a hole in the base of each tin. The jagged edge will be inside. Thread one end of the string through the hole and into one tin. Tie a large knot to prevent it pulling out. Thread the other end

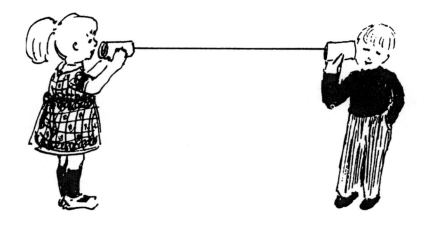

of the string into the second tin and again tie a large knot. Position two children as far apart as the string will allow and give a tin to each. One speaks into her tin while her friend holds his to his ear. Providing the string is held taut, a message will travel along it from one child to the other. Then the roles can be reversed.

LISTENING LIFESAVERS

- Play a game of 'echoes'. You clap once, the child copies you. Clap three times, or what you will.
- Clap a marching or skipping rhythm and the child joins in.
- As a change from clapping, use a percussion instrument or bang the backs of two spoons together.
- For children who are unable to hold an instrument, play the game making mouth noises.
- If you have a group of children, try tapping out the rhythm of someone's name, e.g. 'George' would be one strong tap, 'Henrietta' four short, quick ones. The children must guess the name.

- Tap out the rhythm of a nursery rhyme (This is much more difficult to guess).
- Play a noisy version of 'Follow my Leader'. Whatever sound or rhythm the leader makes, the group must try to imitate.

Playing alone

There are times when every child must play by himself, and this can be a very rewarding experience. He is totally in charge of the pace of the play, and does not have to hurry or wait for his playmates. He is free to let his mind wander off and make intriguing diversions if the mood so takes him. Children with restricted movement are denied energetic play, and, if their energy is in short supply, they are likely to spend quite a lot of time resting. This chapter gives ideas for 'low effort' play for them.

PLAY MATS AND BUSY BOARDS

These are easily obtainable in the shops these days, but for some children the commercial ones may not always be suitable. Perhaps the play mats are too small or the busy boards too large and heavy. They may have unsuitable activities on them, be too cluttered or not sufficiently interesting for the child in question. Even if you already have these items and they seem perfectly satisfactory, perhaps a specially designed one, covered with all the child's favourite sounds and textures may be just what she is secretly wishing for!

Play Mats

Long-lasting

Apart from the ethical question, there is no point in copying a play mat that is already on the shop shelf. It is much more fun to branch out and be adventurous with fabrics and design. I make play mats larger than the normal size and might use an old curtain or even the best part of a duvet cover for the backing. A play mat of generous dimensions gives the child plenty of room to roll about and perhaps 'swim' towards a desirable texture or a toy tied to loops attached near the edges of the mat. I cover the top surface with large areas of textured fabrics and go for maximum impact where colour is concerned. I raid my rag bag and look for velvet, terry towelling, satin, fur fabric, brocade, brightly coloured cotton, corduroy, woolly blanket—even deck chair canvas. I chose the ones that I hope will please the child who will be playing on the mat. (I know one or two who really hate the feel of fur fabric.) Other interesting materials that might come in useful are part of a survival blanket from an outdoor adventure shop and, of course, our old favourite, bubbly plastic used in packaging.

Now for some practical tips:

1. The play mat is likely to make frequent trips to the washing machine, so any fabrics that are not colour-fast or are likely to shrink must go back in the rag bag.

39

2. As the textures are applied in fairly large pieces there is always the possibility that the baby will grab a handful and put it in his mouth. A few spaced out lines of stitching across the patch, as in quilting, will avoid this happening, and will also add strength to the mat.

3. You may want to pad the mat to make it more comfortable to lie on. It must then have an extra backing added so that it is more like a duvet cover, and the padding can be inserted and removed when the cover is washed. A foam plastic bedding roll used by campers might be suitable, or perhaps heavy wadding, cut to size, can be covered with unbleached calico, quilted (to keep it in shape) and finally given a waterproof cover. (For babies who need special support like an air mattress, consult your therapist.)

4. Loops for tying toys to are best attached near the edges of the mat. Knobbly items like rattles are less likely to be rolled on by the baby.

The play mat in the illustration has a further refinement. Handles are firmly attached to the sides so that adults can give the baby a gentle swing.

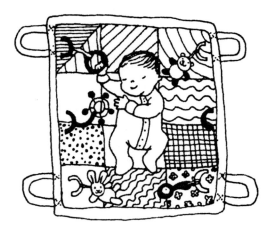

Busy Boards

Long-lasting

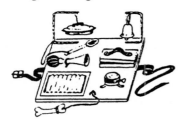

These toy-holders are closely related to the plastic Activity Centres on sale in every toy shop. They have an advantage over their rivals, for they can be tailor-made to fit the needs and interests of a particular toddler or even an older child, who needs his toys to be close at hand. The one illustrated was made for a ten-year-old who had learning difficulties and physical problems. He spent most of his days in a specially adapted wheelchair. His busy board gave plenty of scope for ingenuity. The bicycle bell and the motor horn needed a firm touch to get them going. The other bell and the bone scraper gave a noisy reward for less physical effort. The assortment of noisemakers were mounted on a square of plywood which could be attached to the tray of the boy's wheelchair. With his special busy board in place, he loved to consider himself a one-man band and play along to his favourite pop tunes.

Should you fancy copying the idea, a trip to the DIY store or local ironmongers is sure to produce plenty of attractive noisemakers. For anyone with an electrical bent, the addition of a battery-driven bell or Morse buzzer could turn the busy board into a particularly desirable object, and make its owner the envy of all his friends!

The busy boards I make for babies and toddlers can be tied to cot bars, the backs of wooden chair legs or just rested on the floor. They are made like a cushion cover, or a pillowcase, the size depending on the number of objects I will add to them. I choose a plain fabric which will set off the toys well. Then comes the fun part. The surface of the cover is decorated with all the delights I hope will please the child. These might include a large fabric spot of a contrasting colour sewn to the cover with a squeaker (from a craft shop) behind it, some castanets – from a toy shop, and a bunch of bells, (both firmly attached). I might add some fish grit in a film container, safely encased in a little bag and stitched to the cover, and some large beads to slide along a strip of piping cord—of course, also firmly attached! If there is any room left, I can always add a few loops for tying on favourite rattles, teethers, etc.

41

To make the busy board rigid, a sheet of thick card or hardboard cut to size is inserted inside the cover and the opening is stitched up with a few large tacking stitches—easy to remove if it ever needs a wash. Of course, if the busy board is to be tied in position, tie strings must be sewn to the sides.

FIDDLE TOYS

Whatever our age, it seems there are times when we all love to 'fiddle'—handling something for the sheer pleasure we receive through our sense of touch. Imagine sitting on the beach, sifting the hot, dry sand through your fingers, or twisting an elastic band this way and that. I suppose even stroking the cat might be considered a 'fiddle'! Activities like these are relaxing and give us a pleasant tactile experience. For some children the act of fiddling is not just a way of passing the time. It may help to strengthen their fingers and make them more supple.

Children are inveterate fiddlers and usually find their own favourite objects. Some may not be sufficiently mobile to manage this, and might welcome a ready-made fiddle toy. Here are some suggestions:

A Serendipity of Fiddle Toys

Almost Instant (just allow a little time to collect them all)

Dr Lilli Nielson, Danish expert on the education of visually impaired children

Lilli Nielson has a magic suitcase full of bits and pieces guaranteed to please any child with a passion for fiddling. If you had the chance to lift the lid you would find:

- Four strings of large beads and buttons, joined together at one end to form a tassel.
- Old bed springs with the ends bent in and protected with sticky tape.
- A pliable soap saver with little plastic suckers on the reverse side.
- A bunch of real keys on a strong ring, with a wooden tag to dangle them by.
- An embroidery frame with tracing paper stretched tightly over it, making it like a flat little drum.
- An electric toothbrush holder (without the

brush.) Switch it on and off to experience the pleasant vibration.

- Three long strands of material loosely plaited together, so that a child's fingers can wiggle between the strands.
- A bunch of Bendy drinking straws taped together at the bottom end, so that the bendy part at the mouth end can be twisted about in different directions.
- Large buttons on a loop of elastic.
- Plenty of rattles and tins to shake.

One can imagine any child saying to itself: 'Just let me get at that lot!'

Tactile Bags

Quick

These are made like beanbags, but the contents are chosen for their variety of tactile appeal. Ideally, the covers should be opaque but fairly thin, so that the contents are hidden, but can be easily felt through the fabric. As usual, select items suitable for the child in mind. He may have sharp teeth and plenty of curiosity! If you think there is a possibility he may reveal the contents, go for the safer option and use large items like a teaspoon and a toothbrush, or stick to food like rice and pasta. The bags will have to withstand much squeezing and pinching. It is prudent to sew all seams twice and be fussy about securely closing the gap where you inserted the contents.

Here are some possible fillings to start you thinking:

- A crunched-up potato crisp bag and a ping-pong ball.
- Rice and a few large buttons.
- Two large curtain rings and some dried peas.
- Orange pips and a marble.
- A cotton reel and some coins.

Other possibilities might be some large beads made from plastic or wood, large shells, nuts, lids from Smartie tubes, or everyday objects like a comb, a key, a nylon pan scrubber or a squeaky toy.

An Amorphous Beanbag

Quick

Sylvia O'Bryan, Tutor

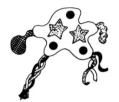

As its name suggests, this beanbag is a wholly unconventional shape. This, of course, is part of its attraction. The body of the beanbag is about the size of a dinner plate, but its shape is anything but circular. Look at the picture and you may be reminded of a 'treasure island' with lots of bays and peninsulas—a much more interesting shape than the conventional square or oblong beanbag.

Add a bunch of ribbons, or a plait or even a small toy to the projecting parts and loosely fill the centre with items from the above list, and the child will love it!

A Manx Feely Cushion

Quick

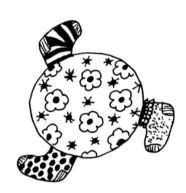

This cushion, like the emblem for the Isle of Man, has three legs. It is a convenient way of keeping three fiddle bags together. The legs are just odd, brightly-coloured baby socks with tactile or noise-making objects inside.

To make it, use a dinner plate as a template and cut out two circles in interesting material, say velvet or fur fabric? Put something tactile or noisy in each of the three socks. Tack across the tops to keep the contents inside. Lay one circle on the table, right side up. Place the socks on it, pointing inwards and with their tops at equal intervals around the circumference. Pin them in place. Cover them with the other circle of material, face downwards, Tack all round the edge of the cushion. Stitch firmly most of the way round it, leaving a gap for turning and stuffing. Turn the cushion the right way out and stuff it with polyester filling, crunchy paper or what you will. Close the gap.

A Tactile Tortoise

Long-lasting

This strange creature was originally made for a little girl with Cerebral Palsy. It soon became her favourite toy. I have made several since the prototype, and all have enticed idle fingers to be busy. One particular success story was with a teenager in the hospital where I then worked. She spent her days mostly in her special chair. She had severe learning difficulties, poor sight and limited movement in her hands. It was difficult to interest her in any of the activities on offer. She only came to life at mealtimes! One day, in desperation, I put a tactile tortoise on her knee. It was quite heavy. I had filled it with chopped up tights for economy! For this girl I now think the weight was important for she could not ignore the strange object resting on her knees. During the singing that concluded the afternoon, we noticed her fingers were beginning to explore all the little cushions on the back of the tortoise. Once she had found the tail filled with marbles, that was it!

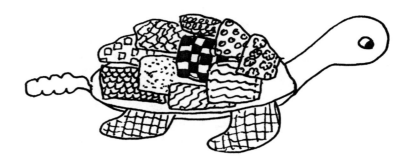

Materials
- Strong material for the body, e.g. tweed, upholstery fabric.
- Thin material in different colours for the little bags that cover the tortoise's back and also form the legs and tail.
- Tactile objects to put in the bags—perhaps some beads, large buttons, crunchy plastic packaging, large curtain rings, fish grit, polyester fibre for a soft feel, some rice (but this won't wash), shells, Smartie tops, a small squeaky toy or a squeaker from a craft shop.
- Scraps of felt for features.
- Filling for the head and body—polyester fibre for a lighter toy.

Method
Using the strong material, cut out the underside of the body. Make it oval and about 30 cm (12") long.

Cut out a second, slightly larger oval. This will be humped up to make the curved back of the tortoise.

Make several small bags in the thinner material—say eight or ten—and put various tactile objects inside. Turn in the tops of the bags and stitch across the opening to keep the contents inside. Arrange the bags on the larger oval, leaving a generous seam allowance round the edge. Machine stitch them in place. (They are supposed to represent the sections on the tortoise's shell!) Make four more bags for the floppy legs and feet (sock shape) and put something tactile in each of them. Tack across the top to prevent the contents from spilling out when you assemble the tortoise. To represent the tail, make a fabric tube. A stretch fabric is best. Stitch across one end and put in about four marbles. Leave space between them so that they can be moved about inside the tail. Tack across the open end.

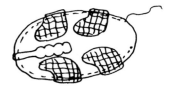

Make a neck and head as in the illustration. Stuff it firmly. Put this part aside while the rest of the tortoise is assembled. On the right side of the underbody pin the legs in position, facing inwards. Pin the tail at the back, but make it point towards where the head will be. Gather round the top section of the body (the shell), so that it will fit the underbody. Pin and tack the shell to the underbody, making sure all the tactile parts—shell segments, legs and tail—are all tucked inside, and then machine stitch most of the way round the tortoise, leaving a gap for turning where the head will go. Turn the whole thing inside out, and you should now have a deflated, headless tortoise! Stuff the body firmly. Push the neck into the opening and sew it securely in place with several rounds of ladder stitching. The head makes a convenient handle and will take a lot of strain. If it tends to flop forward, add extra stitches between the back of the neck and the body until it is as you want it.

Bear in mind the tortoise is not easily washed—especially if you have used pasta or rice in the feely bags! It is best kept as a special treasure for an individual child.

A Chain in a Bottle

Almost Instant

Hettie Whitby,
Teacher

This is a simple but intriguing toy. If you are familiar with Winnie-the Pooh and his friends, you will know the story of Eeyore's birthday present. Pooh and Piglet meant to give him a jar of honey and a balloon, but one got absentmindedly eaten and the other accidentally popped. Eeyore ended up with a bit of damp rubbery rag and an empty honey jar. To his infinite satisfaction he found he could put the popped balloon in the honey jar—and take it out again! His friends left him happily repeating the action over and over again. This toy has the same appeal. Now you see it—now you don't!

The bottle is a discarded plastic one with a handle moulded into it. In its working life it probably contained fabric softener. It is a pretty blue and, of course, the handle makes it easy to hold. The chain can be bought from the local ironmongers or DIY store. The length needed is about twice the height of the bottle. Hettie says a blob of Araldite should stick one end of the chain to the bottom of the bottle. I must confess it did not work for me. Perhaps the bottle was damp inside. I found it was a simple matter to squint down the neck of the bottle, and with some button thread and a long needle, stitch through one side, pick up the end link in the chain and come out the other side. I repeated the process several times, in effect binding the last link in the chain to the bottom of the bottle.

A child can have fun just dropping the chain in and shaking it out again. For some, it is better to go one stage further and tie a cotton reel to the free end of the chain. This makes it easy to hold and prevents it from disappearing totally inside the bottle. Offer this peculiar toy to a child who has just learnt to sit up, or to an inveterate 'fiddler' and you are sure to have a happy and satisfied customer!

JIGSAWS

Jigsaws can certainly be classed as 'low effort' toys and are a useful option for a child with limited energy. Children who enjoy them learn to be

47

observant, to notice colour and shape, to work out if a small piece is part of a face or hand, and if it will fit in a certain space. They will also learn patience and experience a glow of satisfaction when they insert the final piece!

Some children never really take to jigsaws. I have a suspicion that those who are 'jigsaw phobic' once had the unfortunate experience of being totally bewildered by a box full of tiny pieces which they were supposed to fit together. A more considered approach, where the child is offered a puzzle of the right standard of difficulty for him (possibly from the examples below) will usually lead to his enjoyment of this pleasant and restful pastime.

An Inset Puzzle

This type of puzzle can be found in every good toy shop and is perfect for beginners. The pieces are large, easily identifiable and not too numerous. A simple picture is painted on plywood. It might include a tree, a car, a house and a person. Each shape is cut out in one piece. The picture now has gaps where these shapes should fit. It is mounted on a hardboard backing (to prevent the pieces from falling through). The child must return the pieces to their rightful places and so complete the picture.

Most children initially remove the pieces from the puzzle by simply tipping it upside down—a swift and efficient method! For a child who finds this difficult, here are some other ways of removing the pieces:

1. Buy a commercial inset puzzle with a small knob already fitted to each piece.
2. Mount each inset shape on thick cardboard (or use several layers of thinner card,) so that it stands proud of its recess and can be gripped round the edges.
3. Use a shortened golf tee. This makes a useful knob for pulling out a piece, or for replacing a commercial knob that has broken off. Drill a hole the diameter of the golf tee in the piece. If the tee is made of wood, cut it to the right height and glue it in the hole. If it is plastic, poke it in the hole so that the tip just comes out. Rub the

tip with an old spoon which has been heated up. This will melt the plastic and fuse the tee into the hole.

4. Screw a cup hook into each piece. This can be helpful in hooking it out, and can make a useful alternative to a knob.

5. For older children who find removing the pieces difficult, try this popular method. Press a steel drawing pin into each inset piece and use a magnet glued to a handle for pulling it out. Magic! (Remember the safety factor and remove the drawing pins after playtime.)

Now for some simple jigsaw puzzles that can bridge the gap between inset puzzles and the more complicated ones with interlocking pieces.

Christmas Card Jigsaws

Instant

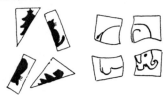

These puzzles can be made in seconds. To make them easier to handle and a little more robust, glue the front of the card to the back. When the glue is dry, cut the card into two, or perhaps four pieces, ready for the child to put back together again. The task is more challenging if two cards with distinctive pictures—say a cat and a tree—are cut up, then muddled together.

A Toy Box Jigsaw

Very Quick

Freda Kim,
Lekotek Korea,
Seoul

From the newsletter of Lekotek (Toy Library) Korea comes an excellent suggestion for recycling as a puzzle, the strong, unwanted cardboard box that originally packaged a toy. The child will have played with the toy, so the picture of it will be familiar. Just cut off the pictorial side of the box and, with a craft knife and a metal ruler (adults only!), neaten the edges and cut the picture into a few bold pieces.

Matchbox Puzzles

Quick

Nylsa do Cunha,
Teacher, Brazil

These puzzles are a novelty for many children. They can be particularly appreciated by children with bandaged hands or who might have to use their feet for play. They can even be manoeuvred by a child using a unicorn head pointer.

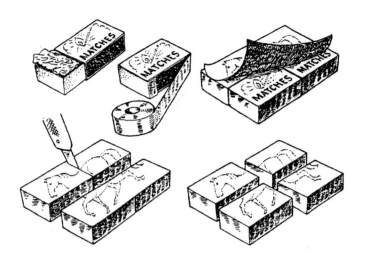

Materials

- Some matchboxes, say four for a very simple puzzle, as illustrated.
- Two pictures, to cover the matchboxes, top and bottom. Choose contrasting ones such as a horse for one side and a woodland scene for the other.
- A few paper tissues.
- Electrician's tape (plastic).
- Possibly some masking tape.

Method

Stuff each matchbox tray with a tissue to give it extra strength, and return it to its cover. Put the matchboxes together and glue one picture over the tops and another over the bottoms. You may find some masking tape round the outside is helpful in holding them in position while you do this. When the glue is dry, separate the matchboxes by cutting between them with a craft knife. Bind round each matchbox with electrician's tape. This serves a dual purpose. It covers the abrasive sides and keeps the trays in place.

A Wooden Push-together Puzzle

Long-lasting

Imagine you have painted a picture on a piece of plywood. Divide it in two by cutting a wavy line down the middle. Before you is a very simple push-together puzzle. If you have the use of a band saw or a jigsaw, you can make these puzzles by the dozen!

Cut as many wiggly lines as appropriate for the child in question. For some, it is sensible to provide a tray for assembling the puzzle. It is easy to jog the pieces out of position, but placing them against the lip of the tray will avoid this frustration.

Two-Piece Jigsaws

Long-lasting

In the early days of the Kingston Toy Library I was watching a little boy try to put together a nine-piece interlocking puzzle. He knew he must join the pieces together, but, like most beginners, he thought he could do this by trying to force them to fit. He had not realised he must look for clues of colour and shape. This cross and frustrated little boy started me thinking. Why not make some simple two-piece puzzles? I experimented with some rectangles of plywood. One was painted yellow, then divided into two with a curved cut as in the illustration. Another, painted red, was bisected with a slightly different curved cut so that one piece from each rectangle would only fit with its partner. With a few more rectangles of different colours added, all the pieces were muddled up. The first child to try out these puzzles soon discovered that she must first pick out the pieces which matched by colour. Then it was easy to fit them together. The puzzles were vastly improved when my friend Audrey Stevenson (a professional toy designer) suggested putting pictures on the reverse side of each pair. Now, as in the illustration, the yellow pair had a banana on the reverse side, a tree on the back of the green one and so on. This made them more interesting and encouraged the child to look for shape as well as colour.

 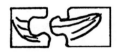

MAKING A SCRAPBOOK

Mary Digby's Special Scrapbook

Quick

Mary was a play specialist in a busy eye hospital. Sometimes the children had one eye bandaged. They could be feeling a little 'frail' and not inclined to join in with group activities. Mary would give such a child a miniature scrapbook made from cheap construction paper. It was about the size of a postcard, and contained just a few pages stitched together in the centre. It could be filled up fairly quickly with small pictures already cut from old Christmas cards, magazines, etc. These were stored in a flat chocolate box, and the child could rootle about among them to make her selection. When provided with a Pritt Stick, she was ready to make her very own scrapbook to take home.

Keeping the box supplied with pictures was a pleasant job for older children who were handy with scissors. Parents, perhaps waiting for their child to come back from Theatre, were also often happy to help.

Making a Scrapbook with a Theme

Quick

Having decided on a theme, in theory the child collects the pictures for her own special book. In practice (for one with restricted movement and limited energy), an adult may need to provide the source of pictures from which she can make her selection.

Of course, the topic for the book will depend on the whim of the child, and her interest for the moment. If ideas are not instantly forthcoming, here are some suggestions:

- A book of colours. Each page contains pictures of one colour. The red page might have a car, a rose, a pair of lips, a bunch of cherries, a red coat ... and so on.
- A book of numbers. Some pictures of one of everything on the first page, perhaps a Christmas tree, a cat, a candle, and a robin; on the next, two carol singers, two rabbits, two holly leaves, etc. (Old Christmas cards are a useful source of pictures for this one!)

- An alphabet book with a picture (or two) selected for its initial letter. A for apple, B for baby, ball, etc.
- Means of transport. There are many imaginative ways of getting from A to B, especially if space travel is included. A book such as this can also be a useful way of helping to bring the world to the child. The artistic and inventive one can use her own contributions as a valuable addition.
- A special interest book—pop stars, the local football club, horses, fashion. The child will certainly have his own ideas for this one!

Finding the Pictures

Christmas (and birthday) cards have already been mentioned as a useful source of supply. There are plenty more. Calendars, gift wrapping-paper, magazines (sometimes available for free from the local hairdresser), specialist journals like the National Geographic Magazine or the RSPB journal 'Birds', travel brochures, mail-order catalogues, newspapers, picture postcards, junk mail, old books (from car boot sales, charity shops.) Once the need is established, it is usually possible to find a source of supply!

A Zigzag Scrapbook

Quick

This is just a variation on the theme, and makes a change from the conventional scrapbook. It is made from stiff paper or card so that it will stand up. It will also fold up and open out like a concertina. Apart from its novelty value, it can be made as long—or as short—as its creator wishes. The one illustrated is like an ordinary scrapbook and is just a collection of pretty pictures. This type of book also lends itself to using a series of related pictures. Take, for example, the topic of 'In the Street'. The zigzag scrapbook could include pictures of shops, cars, buses,

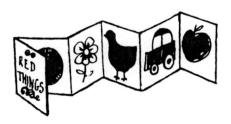

bicycles, a lady with a pram, a fire engine, a lorry, an ambulance, and lots of people. When opened out, the book will show a long picture like a frieze.

Making Miniature Scrapbooks

Quick

When I was a child, the books of stamps had pages of advertisements interleaved between the stamps. My mother would save the empty books for me and I would spend a happy time turning them into picture books for my dolls! This is no longer a practical option, but it is a simple matter for you (or your child?) to stitch together a tiny book made from notepaper. Collect enough miniature pictures, and it could become a scrapbook for a favourite doll or teddy. Who knows where this gentle activity may lead? Provide some slender bridge pencils and a few tiny blank books and the toys are equipped for a game of 'schools'!

THREADING

Threading is a peaceful play activity with many a useful spin-off. It can help to develop nimble fingers and learning skills such as sorting, colour matching, grading and sequencing. It can also encourage concentration and persistence for both of these are needed to produce a string of beads long enough to make a necklace. Leaving aside all these worthy attributes, at some stage in their lives most children really like the action of threading.

First of all, the principle of threading must be understood, and for some children, the simple action of poking the threader through the hole must first be learnt.

- In one toy library they really start from scratch. The volunteers cut plastic rings from washing up liquid bottles. They show the children how to thread these over their hands, to wear on their arms like bangles.
- In an Australian toy library they go one step further, and provide hair curlers for the children to thread on plastic tubing.

- At Lekotek (toy library) Korea they use blocks of wood with holes drilled through them. These are threaded onto a length of dowelling with a rounded tip.
- At our toy library we have a popular toy, which is really intended as a simple button trainer, but it acts equally well as a threading toy. The idea was given to us by Nora Lack, a Paediatric Occupational Therapist. She uses a plastic jar containing plenty of different coloured felt squares. (Packs of small ones are available in craft shops, or you can cut your own.) Some piping cord—say 30 cm (12″)—is threaded through a hole in the lid of the jar and a knot tied on the end to prevent it pulling out. A large button is attached to the other end. The piping cord is unravelled a little way, and the individual strands threaded through the holes in the button and tied together. Next she cuts slots, the right size for the button, in the felt squares which she stores in the jar. Now all the child has to do is delve in the jar for a square and thread it on the string. This action is usually repeated over and over until all the squares are used up.

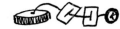

Threading toys are, of course, available from toy shops, but here is an excellent one that is easy to make. It first appeared in the 'Making Toys' programme televised by the BBC several years ago.

The Bee in a Tree

Long-lasting

David Chisnell,
Toy Designer

You will see from the illustration on p. 56 that David cut out a tree in plywood, made holes in the leafy part and attached a chubby bee to buzz in and out; a delightful way of learning to thread.

Not only is this a popular and easily made toy, but there are no pieces to lose. Anyone working in a toy library or hospital where toys are shared will appreciate this point!

Materials
- For the tree, a piece of good quality plywood. For an inferior version, a ping-pong bat with its covering removed can be used.

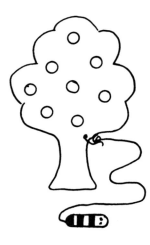

- About 5 cm (2") of dowelling for the bee—or you can use a long, fat macramé bead.
- A length of thin cord for attaching the bee to the tree, say 20–30 cm (8"–12"), or longer, depending on how far the child in question can stretch. Blind cord is a good choice as it will not kink.
- A dab of strong adhesive such as wood glue or Evostick, and a matchstick—for wedging the cord into the bee.
- Sandpaper.
- Paint, and polyurethane varnish for protection.

Method

Assuming you are cutting the tree from plywood, first make a paper pattern. (If you use a ping-pong bat the tree shape is already there.) Fold a sheet of paper lengthwise and draw half the tree against the fold. If you broaden out the base of the tree trunk a little it makes it easier to grasp—a refinement which is not an option if you are using a ping-pong bat. Cut out the shape and open it out. If it is satisfactory, draw round it on the plywood. Drill holes in the leafy part of the tree, large enough for the bee to fly through comfortably. Drill a small hole in the trunk for attaching the cord, and another in one end of the bee (*see* illustration). Round off the other end for the head. Use the sandpaper to smooth all the edges. Paint both sides of the tree green, with a brown trunk. Paint the bee yellow with black stripes and give it a friendly face. Protect all the paint with two coats of polyurethane varnish. Now for the final job of attaching the bee to the tree. Tie one end of the cord to the tree trunk. Squirt some glue in the hole in the bee and insert the free end of the cord. A needle is helpful in feeding it in. Fix it firmly in place with a small wedge cut from a matchstick and coated with adhesive.

The Happy Tree

Long-lasting

Inspired by the toy above I made a threading tree for a very bright little girl with brittle bones. A challenging and light-weight toy was required. My tree differed from David's in that separate pieces (attachments) in the shapes of birds, butterflies, flowers or

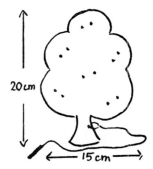

fruit, were threaded onto it. There were two holes in each attachment, and corresponding pairs were drilled in the tree. A shoelace acted as the threader and was used to 'stitch' the attachments to the tree with an 'up one hole and down the other' movement.

Materials
- A small piece of three ply, say 20 cm × 15 cm (8" × 6").
- A round shoelace.
- Sandpaper.
- Paint.
- Polyurethane varnish.

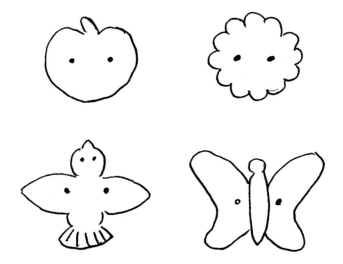

Method
It is always a wise move to start with a paper pattern. As with the 'Bee in a Tree', fold the paper in half, draw half the tree, cut it out and open the paper out. Follow the same method for the attachments—butterflies, birds, fruit or flowers. Transfer the paper shapes to the plywood, cut them out, and sandpaper the edges. Drill small pairs of holes exactly the same distance apart in all the attachments and in pairs on the tree. Drill one hole in the trunk for the shoelace. Paint all the pieces, protect your work with polyurethane varnish and tie on the shoelace.

Making a Necklace

Now we come on to what children call 'proper threading'. For this activity to be free from frustration and irritability, it is often necessary to do a little preparation.

1. *Provide a stable container for the beads*. This is particularly important for children in bed where small items are easily lost among the covers, and for those who are unable to bend down and retrieve dropped beads. A plastic cereal bowl is suitable, but it is light and easily knocked over. Stabilise it on the bed table or tray with a blob of Blu-tac or a loop of masking tape squashed flat and attached to the bottom of the bowl.

2. *Make sure the threader will slip easily through the bead and out the other side*. A round shoelace will often do the job, but for larger beads a splendid threader can be made from a short length of polypropylene clothes line. This is the thin one (without a wire core) which is used for whirly lines. It is stiff enough to poke through the bead and be grasped easily as it comes out the other side. Jewellers sell nylon threaders with a stiff wire end. These are excellent for older children, who are interested in making their own jewellery.

3. *Supply beads that are right for the age and capability of the child*. Brightly-coloured wooden beads can be bought at most toy shops. Square ones will not roll away and are easier to hold than the round ones. Attractive beads for older children can often be found at charity shops and car boot sales.

Home-made Beads

1. Drinking Straws
Here is an instant activity which pleased my own children when they were little. We held a bunch of drinking straws over a cereal bowl and cut them into short lengths of about 1 cm. The cereal bowl caught them as they fell. Threaded onto pipe cleaners they made excellent bracelets for the dolls and teddies!

Using a blunt needle and double cotton (so that the needle did not constantly become unthreaded!), they also made attractive necklaces.

2. Paper Beads
These have been around for so long that they maybe considered 'traditional'. Some parents of my generation may have forgotten to pass on the simple technique for making them, so here it is. Directions are given with an adult in mind, but this is also an excellent activity for older children with nimble fingers.

Materials
- A knitting needle. Its gauge determines the size of the hole in the bead.
- Some non-glossy paper.
- PVA adhesive.
- Paints for the decoration.
- Polyurethane varnish.

Method
Tear the paper into strips against the edge of the table or a ruler. The longer and wider the strip the larger the finished bead will be. After a few trials you will find the right size for the child in question. Wrap one end of the strip round the knitting needle, then apply the PVA adhesive and continue to roll up the strip as tightly as possible. Try not to get adhesive on the knitting needle or the finished bead will be difficult to slide off. You should now have a well-formed cylindrical bead. Put it aside to dry out, and make some more. When all are dry, decorate them and protect with polyurethane varnish.

If you prefer a rounder bead, make the strips of paper taper at one end like a pennant. Start rolling up from the wide end. If you use wallpaper, the beads will turn out chunkier and you will need a shorter strip.

3. Bamboo Beads
These unusual beads are easily made from short lengths cut from garden canes. I made the first

ones from the bits and pieces left over from the 'Bamboo Mobile' described on p. 24. When painted and varnished, the finished beads are very attractive, light and strong and have a sizeable hole in the centre. Children love them and any little girl who makes them into a necklace for herself is likely to receive orders from all her friends! I think they are well worth the time it takes to make them.

Materials
- Bamboo garden canes, say two, but of course it depends on the number of beads you want to make.
- A knitting needle.
- Sandpaper.
- Paint. Acrylic is best, poster will do.
- Polyurethane varnish.
- A threader and a box to hold the beads.

Method
Remove the waxy layer from the outside of the bamboo with a craft knife. Scrape away from yourself. Next, saw the bamboo into short lengths of about $2\frac{1}{2}$ cm (1"). Avoid the joints and any uneven parts. Clean out the pith in the centre with a knitting needle. Sandpaper each bead for a really smooth surface. Now for the fun part! Paint each bead as your fancy dictates, and protect your designs with polyurethane varnish. When dry, package them in an attractive box and add the threader.

A handcrafted set of beads like these can make a very special and unusual present.

Some Threading Lifesavers

- Try this simple activity which you probably enjoyed in your youth. If you know the child you have in mind has reached the stage of being able to handle a needle with safety, provide her with a box of buttons and a blunt needle. Thread the needle and pull the thread through until the ends are level. (Using the thread double will avoid the needle becoming unthreaded every five seconds!) Tie a button on the end of the thread to stop the ones the child threads from falling off, and let her loose with the button box.

- Thread up squares of toast and hang them up for the birds!
- Make a necklace from pasta shapes.
- If it is possible to obtain the inner cylinders from a shop cash till, these make excellent large beads for beginners to thread. I find friendly check-out girls are pleased to save them for a good cause! They can be used just as they are, or the plastic ones can be decorated with Humbrol Enamel (sold in small tins for painting models). The cardboard ones can be coloured with felt pens or paint. A coat of polyurethane varnish will add to their durability.

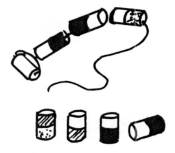

See also
A Straw Dancing Dolly, p. 129.

MAZES

Open any children's comic and you are certain to find a maze somewhere among the pages. This simple puzzle seems to appeal to anyone who can ably guide a pencil. You will even find them in puzzle books aimed at adults. Anyone who can hastily draw a satisfactory one will have a sure means of amusing a child during a long wait or on a boring journey.

A puzzle maze in its simplest form is just a path, which wanders from one side of the page to the other. The object, of course, is to find the route from the beginning of the maze to the end without crossing a line. Here and there another path will lead from the main one, but this could be a 'blind alley'. Anyone guiding his pencil along such a false trail will have to retrace his steps.

Drawing a Maze on Paper

To make a rectangular maze as illustrated, first mark the start and the finish. With your pencil at 'Start',

61

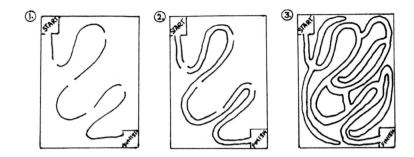

faintly draw a line meandering across the page until it reaches 'Finish'. (If you do not make the line firm at this stage you can easily rub it out if you wish to make any changes.) You now have one side of the path planned out. Rub out small gaps in the line for the blind alleys that can be added later. Draw the other side of the path parallel to your first line, and again leave the odd gap here and there. Now draw the blind alleys leading from the gaps in the main path. Make them as long as possible, so that they are not too obvious. Perhaps one or two might be a short cut.

A Circular Maze

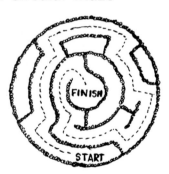

One this shape is easy to contrive, but more difficult to solve.

1. With a pair of compasses, lightly draw several concentric circles—like a target. Make as many rings as you want.

2. Mark the starting point on the outer line and, of course, 'Home' will be inside the smallest circle. The object will be to follow a path to the bull's eye in the centre. Draw a faint pencil line to indicate the direction of the path (dotted in the illustration). This must wander through gaps from one circle to another, sometimes crossing back to the previous one, and meandering all over the target area.

3. Block off the blind alleys with firm lines—not too close to the main path so that it is not instantly obvious that they lead nowhere. Rub out the faint line you drew to indicate the route. You now have gaps in the circles where the path passes through them. Draw darkly over

the remaining parts of the circles. I have done a scribble over mine to represent a hedge from above!

A Maze in a Flan Tin

*Quick to make,
but a long-lasting game*

A cardboard circle is cut to fit the base of the flan tin. On this a maze is drawn, and the lines are covered with string—to make little walls. The object is to guide a marble through the maze by gently tilting the flan tin this way and that—a feat which calls for concentration and skill.

Materials
- A flan tin.
- Some fairly sturdy cardboard—the back of a writing pad will do.
- A small amount of ribbon or tape.
- String or piping cord. A thick one makes it easier to keep the marble on track.
- A marble.

Method
While you are on the job, it is a good idea to make several mazes, graded in difficulty, to fit in the bottom of the flan tin. Cut circles of cardboard, using the bottom of the tin as a template. Check that they fit snugly in the tin before going to the trouble of making the mazes. It is a wise move to attach a tab of ribbon or tape to the rim of each circle. This makes it easy for the child to lift it out if he wants to replace it with another. As with the circular paper maze, work out the path for the marble to take, and draw the route with parallel lines. Remember that when you edge the path with string it will become slightly narrower. Next apply the string. Measure the length you need for a section, squirt a line of PVA adhesive along the maze line, then press the string onto it. I find this less messy than applying the adhesive to the string. Without disturbing the string, gently roll the marble along the route to check that it can move through the maze without getting stuck. Leave the adhesive to dry properly.

Beginners appreciate a coloured track for the marble to follow. Leave the blind alleys plain.

A Cloth Marble Maze

Long-lasting

This simple toy has novelty value. There is nothing like it available in the shops! It is light and unbreakable—so can easily be sent through the post. It can be made easy or more difficult according to the need of the moment. There are no parts to lose, so it can make a useful diversion on the coach journey to school or in the car, AND it can go through the washing machine when it becomes grubby!

It consists of two layers of cloth stitched together to form channels. The challenge for the child is to squeeze a marble, or a bead, through the channels and make it travel from point A to point B. The route may be from the edge to the centre of a fairly simple spiral as in Illustration 1 or it might wander over the area of the fabric as in a paper maze. Illustration 2 shows an X-ray view of an easy maze. The dotted lines indicate the stitching. To make the channels show up clearly, I have shaded in the blocked off areas. If you want the marbles visible at the beginning and end of the maze, follow the directions for the colour maze below and make net curtain 'windows' at the start and finish. Illustration 3 shows an elementary colour maze. In play, a red, blue, green and yellow marble starts at the centre of the maze and must be squeezed through the channels until each one reaches its appropriate corner.

1.

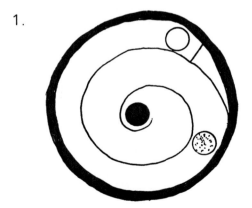

2.

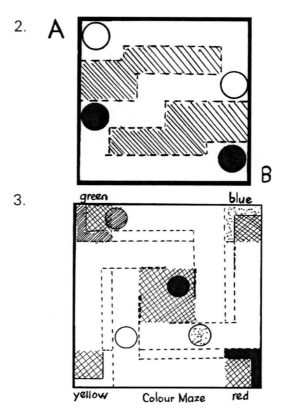

3.

Materials
- Scrap paper for planning the maze.
- Fabric for the cloth part. Unbleached calico is ideal.
- A marble or bead—maybe more then one.
- Nylon net if you want windows as in Illustration 3. If you prefer, you can make the whole of the top layer of the maze in net. This makes the passage of the marble through the channels visible as well as well as tangible.
- Bias binding to make a frame round the edge. This keeps the marbles inside the maze and adds a touch of colour.

Method
First plan your maze on paper. Make sure the channels are just wide enough for the marbles to travel freely without getting stuck. The only sure

way of checking this is to sew some experimental channels on two layers of scrap cloth and try them for size. I have a favourite ruler which is just the right width to mark out a channel for an average marble. Next draw your maze to scale on the underside of the bottom layer of the sandwich. Pin both layers together. Stitch the channels, following your pencil lines. Put in the marble(s) and sew bias binding all round the edge of the maze.

The simple colour-sorting maze in Illustration 3 is made slightly differently from the other two. The top layer of calico is backed with nylon net curtaining. The squares in the corners are stitched in the appropriate colours, using a close zigzag stitch on the sewing machine. The calico is carefully cut away from the squares, leaving the net exposed. This top layer· is then backed with calico and the channels stitched as indicated by the dotted lines. Four marbles of the appropriate colours are inserted before adding the border of bias binding.

These mazes were so popular with some of the children at the toy library that I found myself elaborating on the idea. In my rag bag I found some pictorial fabric which seemed full of possibilities. From one piece, I cut out an apple tree and a basket and contrived a maze where small red beads had to be squeezed down the channels leading from the tree at the top of the maze to the basket waiting below. Further inspiration came from a picture of a boy who appeared to be singing. It was a simple matter to stitch him at the end of the maze and put an oval shape at the beginning for a plate. This time bead 'food' was manipulated from the plate to the boy's mouth! ('Tops' for child appeal!)

MAKING USE OF MAGNETS

I know a house where the front of the fridge is decorated all over with brightly coloured plastic magnetic letters. They seem to have a magnetic attraction for the family, for they are frequently being rearranged to spell out messages and jokes.

Bought magnetic toys in their many different forms seem to be popular with everyone from preschool to retirement age. But they can be of special value to children with restricted movement for they will stay where they are put.

Magnetic travel toys can, of course, be bought at motorway services stations. Large toy shops stock magnetic letters and toys like magnetic bricks and shapes for making patterns. Joke shops can sometimes be a good source for magnetic novelties. Even with these sources of supply, it may be difficult to find a toy which has just the right appeal for the child in question. Luckily, it is a simple matter to apply magnetic properties to an existing toy or even to invent a new one to please a special child. A home-made magnetic fishing game is always a winner and suggestions for making one are given on p. 71.

Magnetic play

Children who cannot reach far or who must play on a bed table or the tray of their wheelchair appreciate a toy which will stay where it is put! Add magnetic properties to one, and it is less likely to be pushed out of reach, dropped or lost among the bedclothes. There are only two basic requirements for this kind of play—a metal surface and toys with magnets attached!

The play surface need not be a problem. The front of the fridge has already been mentioned, but for children for whom this is not an option, perhaps they may already have a metal play board belonging to another toy. Failing that, an ordinary tin tray or a metal baking tray or tin will often answer the purpose. (Some are made from an alloy and a magnet will not stick to them so 'try before you buy!')

Now for the magnets.

Magnetic tape is sold as a ribbon with an adhesive backing. It is excellent for attaching to light card toys and can even be stitched to cloth—an important point if there is any danger of a child trying to eat it!

Bar and disc magnets are more powerful and ideal for mounting on plywood or thick card. These come in many strengths, shapes and sizes. Some small ones for making fridge magnets are usually available at craft shops. Magnets in several varieties which are used for school scientific purposes can be bought by post from educational suppliers, *see* p. 184, and Dowling Magnets, p. 185. DIY shops can also be a useful source of supply. These magnets seem to hold their magnetism longer than the tape, and are easy to apply to toys or pictorial card shapes—perhaps to use with a metal board for story telling. Use a strong glue in a tube, like Evostick. (Read the directions on the box!)

To apply a magnet to a shiny plastic toy, it may be necessary to scratch a small area of the plastic with a file or coarse sandpaper to give the glue a chance to stick to it.

Magnetic Toys

Quick

Deborah Jaffé,
Toy Designer

Way back in 1975 Deborah wrote a delightful little book called *Magnetic Board Toys*. It was published by the then National Toy Libraries Association and sadly is no longer in print. Deborah has given me permission to pass on some of her ideas.

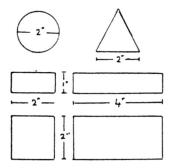

A magnetic mosaic
From 4 mm ply or thick card, make a selection of geometric shapes—squares, circles, triangles, rectangles using the dimensions suggested in the illustration. Given plenty of pieces, these can be used to make a variety of pictures and patterns. Colour the shapes. Acrylic paint is best, but poster paint or felt pens will do. It is wise to protect the painted surface with a coat of polyurethane varnish or cover it with clear sticky-backed plastic. Cut the magnetic tape into pieces and stick them to the back of each shape. Use several small pieces rather than one large one—or even a strip—because the adhesion to the metal board will be better.

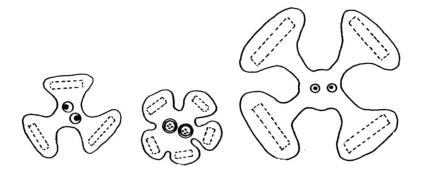

A creepy crawly

Consult the illustration and take your pick! Each one is made from two pieces of material with magnetic tape sandwiched in between. Choose lightweight material like cotton, voile, poplin or nylon. Indicate the eyes on the top piece. These might be snap-on safety eyes from a craft shop, buttons (firmly attached), felt (stuck and stitched), or embroidered. On the bottom piece stitch magnetic tape to the inside of the feet—*see* dotted lines on the illustration.

Put the pieces right sides together and pin. Stitch most of the way round the outside, leaving a small gap for turning. Turn right side out and close the gap (oversew).

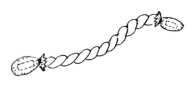

A creepy crawly worm

Make this from a short length of piping cord—say 15 cm (6"). Sew magnetic tape to the ends and, for safety's sake, cover it with little bags stitched to the piping cord.

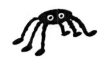

A spider with six feet

Use three slightly longer pieces of piping cord than for the worm. It is wise to tackle the magnetic feet first, before the cord tends to unwind. Stitch a small piece of magnetic tape to every end. Cover the feet with little bags as above. Overlap the cords in the middle and stitch them together. Splay out the legs for realism! Make a body from two ovals of black felt and top stitch them together to cover the cords where they intersect. Sew on tiny beads for eyes or indicate them with French knots.

Some More Ideas

Push-together puzzles (see p. 50.)

These puzzles are ideal for magnetic play. The pieces just need to be pushed together in the right order to make up the picture. In one hospital where I worked, we had an ancient and unattractive brown metal cupboard which I brightened up with several small, wooden push-together puzzles. On Friday evenings I muddled them up ready for our Monday morning visitors. Over the weekend the cleaning lady would amuse herself by putting them all back together again. Like some of the children, she must have found them irresistible—or perhaps she thought she was helping to tidy up!

For a quick push-together puzzle all you need is a Christmas card. Stick the front to the back to make it stiffer. Wait for the glue to dry, then, with a crooked line cut the card into pieces—perhaps just two for a beginner, more for a child who is used to jigsaws. Cut the magnetic tape into squares and apply several to the backs of all the pieces. (As mentioned above, several small pieces grip the metal surface better than one long strip.)

For long-lasting puzzles use ply. A picture merely stuck on may be 'picked' at the edges and the puzzle soon ruined. It is best to paint the picture directly onto the wood. With a fretsaw cut wavy lines to divide it into the number of pieces you want, smooth the edges with sandpaper, apply magnetic tape or disc magnets and finish off with a protective coat of polyurethane varnish over the picture.

A new life for animal templates

At the toy library we have plywood sets of animals, methods of transport, etc. for the children to draw round. Over time these become very messy with all the lines made by felt pens that have accidentally strayed over the surface. They are soon recycled as desirable objects for story telling! I paint over the scribbles, protect the shapes with polyurethane varnish and apply squares of magnetic tape to the backs. I now have a collection of animals, cars, lorries, vans and aeroplanes to put on my magnetic story board as required.

Magnetic Games which use Wire Paper Clips

Quick

These are intended for older children, unlikely to come to harm from any of the materials used. If there is a lively toddler in your household wait until his bedtime before trying them out. Stray paper clips have been known to turn up in the most unexpected places like up noses or in ears.

Two fishing games
Cut out a fish shape in thin card, attach a paper clip to its mouth, and it is ready to be caught by a magnet on a string. If you want your fish to float in a bowl of water or in the bath, cut them from thin plastic, such as the lid of an ice cream box.

For younger children (and those of unknown habits) I use daisy clips. These are obtainable from office stationers and consist of a disc of metal like a daisy (which should sit on top of a document) and two little legs which poke through the pages and then splay out to keep them firmly together. I make the fish fairly large, cut each shape out twice in thin card and paint both halves. In one, I insert a daisy clip where I judge the eye should be and hammer it really flat. Another daisy clip goes in the other half. I place this one so that it will not lie over the first. I want the finished fish to be as flat as possible and if one clip ends up on top of the other they can form a bump. Next, the halves are united with a strong adhesive and I hold the edges together with clothes pegs until the glue has set. If the fish are intended to be used many times, it is worth taking the trouble to cover them with clear sticky-backed plastic or to give them a coat of polyurethane varnish to protect the paint and make them easily wiped clean.

Apparently toys and games making use of paper clips and magnets have been around for many years in the Far East, but it was only recently that I saw some which had been made for children in Korea. Starting with clear plastic containers like water bottles and trays for holding portions of food, the creators of these ingenious games then placed some wire paper clips inside. Using a magnet held to the outside of the container the challenge was to guide the paper clips in a controlled manner and deposit them on a target inside. This principle can have other applications. Freda Kim, Director of Toy Libraries in Korea, tells me of a similar toy she makes from a large, flat chocolate box. She draws a roadway layout on the inside of the base of the box and sprinkles in a few paper clips to represent cars. Holding magnets against the underside of the box, two children can direct the paper clip traffic according to the Highway Code—or more likely, they will play 'Cops and Robbers' and go for pile-ups and crashes!

Inspired by these simple toys, I collected together some cardboard, paper and felt pens, a few clear plastic containers, a packet of magnets and a box of paper clips. Just to show you some of the possibilities, here are the results of my evening's experiments:

1. I began with a roadway similar to, but a little larger than the one made by Freda Kim. Mine was intended to be a game for two little boys, who were able to sit at opposite sides of a table. The game would lie between them. A roadway snaked its way over the surface of a sheet of thick card. There were crossroads, roundabouts, hairpin bends and cul-de-sacs, houses, shops, a petrol station, a car park and a school to visit. In play, the card roadway was supported on two thick books, and the children were supplied with old wooden rulers which had bar magnets glued to the ends. Paper clips were wrapped in short strips of gummed paper and decorated—to make them distinguishable from each other and look

more like cars. When these were placed on the roadway and the magnets held under it, they could be guided around the roadway at the whim of the children. It is satisfactory to report that this simple toy was very popular and led to lots of conversation and imaginative play.

It would be easy for some children to make a roadway for themselves. It might even be drawn to represent a map of their district. This flat type of puzzle could also be drawn as a river and fish substituted for cars and, of course, it could also be made as a maze puzzle (p. 62) or a racing circuit.

2. Next, I tried some puzzles in containers. The advantage here was that the paper clips were encased within the container and could not be dropped or lost among the bedclothes.

First to hand was a clear plastic water bottle. It was clean and dry inside. I put in some coloured wire paper clips, and screwed on the cap. Taking a strip of paper and using felt pens to match the colours of the paper clips, I made some evenly spaced spots in a row. These were bound in place with Sellotape against the outside of the bottle. When, the bottle was lying on its side, the spots could be seen from above. The bottle was shaken a little so that the paper clips were separated out. Holding the bottle steady with one hand and with a magnet in the other, I contacted a paper clip and guided it over the surface of the bottle until it was just above the spot that matched its colour. When the magnet was taken away from the side of the bottle the paper clip dropped neatly onto its target. I continued like this until all the paper clips had found their mark.

3. A food container with a transparent plastic lid from the supermarket came next. It was soon transformed into a simple puzzle. This time the paper clips had to be dropped into the screw top lid from a plastic bottle of milk. Here I discovered a technical hitch! I attached the milk bottle

top (upside down so that it was like a small dish) to the bottom of the inside of the container with a blob of Blu-tac. It was only after I had put in the paper clips and Sellotaped the lid in place that I discovered the toy would not work! The paper clips soon became trapped under the edge of the milk bottle top and the magnet was powerless to move them. The solution was easy. I removed the lid and made sure that the Blu-tac covered the whole of its surface, leaving no gaps.

4. Next came a puzzle in an ice cream tub. A simple colour-matching puzzle could soon be made using the different coloured screw tops from plastic milk bottles—full cream, semi-skimmed, and skimmed! Making sure that this time there would be no gaps under the lids, I positioned them on the floor of the ice cream tub with Blu-tac, and cut down the sides of the tub to about 5 cm (2") high. If left untrimmed, the magnet was not near enough to the paper clips to lift and drag them efficiently. I then put in the coloured paper clips to match the lids. I covered the top of the tub with some thick polythene from one of my husband's Orienteering map cases held firmly in place with Sellotape.

CRAFTS AND HOBBIES

Sometimes, at an early age, a child will show a passionate interest in a particular subject—usually football! For those unable to be involved in such physical activities, collecting information about a hero, and if lucky, cheering at his matches may be the nearest they are able to get to the action. For some, even this active audience participation may not be an option. Alternative ways of using leisure time must be offered.

If your child is growing out of the toy stage and wanting a new diversion—one that might possibly lead to a life-long interest—perhaps something on the following list will suggest a starting point. To describe all the crafts and hobbies in detail would probably make a book in itself, so I have confined myself to the basics and, where possible, have suggested sources of more information. I set out to try to find a craft or hobby for every letter of the alphabet and have nearly succeeded! If I have forgotten your favourite, never mind. You are the expert and can take it from there!

A *Acting*

See Finger Puppets, p. 140 and Glove Puppets, p. 147, What to do with a Shoe Box, p. 179, The dolls' house can easily become a tiny theatre.

B *Bead craft*

An instruction book and a wide variety of beads are available from the Craft Depot, Somerton Business Park, Somerton, Somerset, TA11 6SB. Tel: 01458 272 932 E-mail: craftdepot@aol.com

They make a small charge for the catalogue. Minimum order is £10, so get together with your friends!

See also
Threading, p. 58.
Fimo, p. 77.

Bird Watching
For a catalogue of bird tables, nesting boxes, bird feed etc. and an excellent little book called

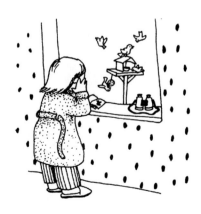

The Birds in your Garden contact the Royal Society for the Protection of Birds, The Lodge, Sandy, Bedfordshire, SG 19 2DL, Tel. 01767 680 551, www.rspb.org.uk. A window bird feeder that attaches to the window pane with suction pads is available from OXFAM, some garden centres and pet shops.

Perhaps enquire at the local public library for possible bird watching groups in your area.

Clay

This is an advance on modelling with playdough (*see* p. 175) and requires a little more manual strength. Newclay is a non-brittle, non-toxic clay that can be hardened without a kiln. The Newclay Activity Pack gives directions on how to make thumb pots, tiles, jewellery and 3D models. Available from Hope Education, Orb Mill, Huddersfield Road, Oldham, Lancashire, OL4 2ST, Tel: 0161 633 6611; E-mail, orders@hope-education.co.uk. They also supply modelling tools and grey and terracotta clay.

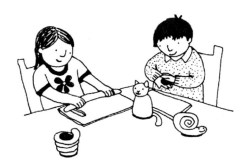

Collections

According to the interests of the child. Some popular ones are pictures and memorabilia of pop or sports stars, stamps, shells, pressed leaves or even colourful plastic rubbers in a multiplicity of shapes.

Computers

Approach an expert!

Crochet
Ask Grandma perhaps for initial instruction. Wool shops stock patterns for the efficient and there are likely to be books in the public library.

D *Dolls*
See p. 127.

E *Embroidery*
I find children usually need to be inspired to begin this absorbing hobby by following the example of another person—usually a friendly and patient adult. There are many books and magazines to suggest stitches and projects, and boxed starter kits are on sale in many toy shops.

See also
Sewing, p. 81.

F *Fimo*
This colourful modelling medium is useful for older children. It is similar to Plasticine, but can be fired in the oven. It is widely available at craft shops etc., and is excellent for making beads, small models (people?), dolls house accessories, etc.

G *Gardening*
If you need help with this one, there are gardening books galore in every public library.

See also
Growing Things, p. 108.

H *Horse riding*
Contact 'Riding for the Disabled', Avenue R, National Agriculture Centre, Kenilworth, Warwickshire CV8 2LV.

I *Instruments*
For a child with even modest musical talents, making music with other people can be intensely satisfying.

A percussion instrument, such as a drum, (saucepan and wooden spoon?), tambourine or bell shakers, makes a good starting point. The child only needs to concentrate on the rhythm. When it comes to more complicated music making, provide a proper instrument if possible, not a toy version. For example, there are toy wooden xylophones on the market, but the notes are not always tuned correctly and it is not easy to pick out a recognisable melody. A well made, more expensive version from a music shop will make a pleasant sound and eventually be a joy to play—and listen to! For children with small hands a tin whistle may be easier to play than a recorder. Their fingers must be able to cover the holes.

J *Jewellery making*

See also
Threading, p. 58; Bead Craft, p. 75; Fimo, p. 77.

K *Kites*
Write to Brookite Limited, Brightly Mill, Okehampton, Devon, EX20 1RR Tel: 01837 53315; E-mail: HYPERLINK mailto:sales@brookite.com. They supply small kites, wind socks, and 'Wind things', by mail order, also materials for making your own.

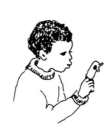

Knitting
Initial instruction needs to be from a patient adult. Once the child has learnt to plain and purl, cast on and off, increase and decrease, an exciting range of patterns is available at every wool shop.

See also
Finger Puppets, p. 141.

L *Letter writing* – either by e-mail or 'snail mail'.
'Write Away' is an unique pen friend scheme for children aged 8–18, who have any kind of disability or special need. For a small charge it offers a Quarterly Newsletter in print, cassette, Braille and

other services. Tel: 020 8964 4225; E-mail: pen-friends@writeaway.demon.co.uk

 Models

In the early stages these are often made from junk—cardboard cartons, cotton reels, etc., all glued together to make the desired object. Later on, models from kits like Lego, K'nex, or Airfix come into their own. For children who can use scissors, there are many cut-out cardboard models on the market including a complete dolls' house designed by Maureen Roffey.

Music making

Children with musical talent may be able to join a local youth choir or play in a children's orchestra or band. These are usually listed in the local public library, or look in the local press for reviews of concerts, attend the next one and see if the standard and type of music presented is what you are looking for.

 Night sky observations

Consult an expert!

◖ *Origami*

Learn the basics from a friend, then look in books for more ideas.

▐ *Papier mâché*

If you fancy some messy play, go for this! A recipe for paste and notes on the technique can be found on p. 172.

Pebble painting

If you are fortunate enough to live near the sea or a shallow river, you may find a smooth pebble with a flat base that would be perfect for converting into a paperweight. Wash it, dry it, paint it, coat it with polyurethane varnish, stick felt to the base (to stop it from scratching the furniture) and you have a perfect paper weight.

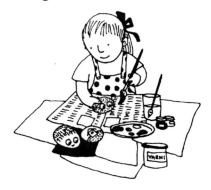

Photography
There is likely to be an expert close at hand—family or neighbour—who will be happy to give advice if needed.

Playdough
See p. 176 for recipes. Playdough is ideal for a play session, then it can be stored in a jar or plastic bag in the fridge until the next occasion. It will happily last for about a week. Salt dough, very similar, but without the added oil, can be moulded, baked, painted and varnished to make a variety of decorations. Try the public library for books of ideas.

Printing
Anyone can make a hand print—sometimes with a little help! This is a simple way of showing a child

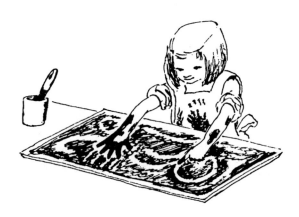

how to transfer paint from one source to another. The little girl in the illustration is having a real 'hands on' experience, and her paint, thickened with a little flour and water paste, is spread over a tray. For more information on printing, *see* p. 174.

Ⓠ *Quilling*

This is a hobby for the nimble fingered. Very narrow strips of coloured paper are coiled and glued to card to make attractive designs and pictures. An instruction book, tools and equipment are available from the Craft Depot, *see* Bead Craft, p. 75.

Quilting

A needlework technique involving small running stitches. It is suitable for older girls.

Ⓡ *Raffia work*

I have not noticed coloured raffia in the shops for some time, but it is included here for the sake of the letter R!

The only kind readily available is sold at garden centres for tying up plants. I have seen it used to make dolls, like corn dollies or the woollen ones described on p. 128. I have a set of tablemats lovingly worked with raffia over string, using 'lazy squaw' stitch. You may remember this from your youth.

Ⓢ *Sewing*

There are many books on the subject, but I think plastic canvas deserves a special mention. It is sold by the sheet and can be cut to size. When covered in wool (cross or tent stitch) it looks very attractive. It is washable and makes beds, chairs, cookers, chests of drawers etc. for the dolls' house. It is ideal for young children and beginners, and the more able can use a smaller mesh size to produce beautiful photograph frames, boxes etc. *See also* the Mother Duck snapper puppet p. 146. This pattern—without the beak—stitched in the appropriate colours will also make a badger, fox, etc. Instruction books and materials are available from the Craft Depot, *see* Bead Craft, p. 75.

Stamp collecting

This can be a perfect hobby for a child who is interested in geography, history, art, nature and people. It is also a sociable one, for good collections are added to by swapping.

See also

Bringing the World to the Child, p. 113.

Swimming

Contact your local swimming bath. Many are equipped with hoists, etc. which are necessary for some children and they may have special sessions when the Baths are not crowded.

Stencilling

Sets of stencils are easily available on the High Street and can be used for many purposes—such as making book marks, gift cards, friezes or decorating posters. Used with care, a good result is guaranteed.

T *Tie dying*

This is a popular craft in schools and nearly always gives good results. The trick is to do the tying very tightly, so that the die cannot penetrate the crunched-up area. It is a fun technique for decorating handkerchiefs, tee shirts, or even for making white pillowcases more decorative.

Tracing

This can be a popular occupation with children who delight in careful, neat occupations. One of the snags can be that, if the tracing paper moves a little, it may be difficult for the child to reposition it accurately over the picture. One way of avoiding this is to put the picture to be traced inside a greaseproof paper bag, and fold the bag to fit snugly round the picture. (Greaseproof bags have not been totally replaced by plastic ones. They are still around in small shops. If desperate, you can always make your own from a sheet of greaseproof paper readily available for cooking purposes.)

Weaving

I have recently discovered stick weaving—a simple technique which can be a useful introduction to the weaver's craft. It is particularly suitable for children with limited reach. It requires lengths of thin dowel, about 15cm (6") long, rounded at one end and with a small hole drilled in the other. The warp thread is threaded through this and becomes double. In action, the pegs (two to start with) are held parallel to each other in one hand, with the warp dangling down. The ends of the warp are tied together to prevent the finished weaving from sliding off. With the other hand, wool is wound between the sticks in a figure-of-eight movement. When they are partly covered with wool, the work is slid gently over the string, being careful to leave some weaving still on the sticks to help keep them parallel. Children can become addicted to this simple weaving and will produce strips of it! Short lengths can be converted into caterpillars, coiled into snail shapes or arranged as a child's initial and stitched to a treasure bag as an impressive means of identification. Longer lengths can be coiled and stitched into mats or coasters. For children with larger hands, wider weaving, suitable for belts or joining together for a flat surface, can be made by holding say five sticks in one hand. For full information and equipment for stick weaving, peg loom weaving and cord making, contact Mrs Maureen Preen, Craft Products, Ivy House, Deep Cutting, Pool Quay, Welshpool, Powys, SY21 9LJ
Tel. 01938 590 533.

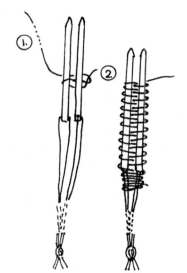

PLAYING ALONE LIFESAVERS

On the Practical Side

- Give the child some means of signalling for help if desperately required. Perhaps the Ship's Bell on p. 30.
- Devise a way of organising toys so that they don't all get lost among the bedclothes, (*see* Play Cushion, p. 8) Some parents use a peg bag as a toy-holder, others pin a carrier bag to

the sheet. (The latter can be an excellent way of disposing of rubbish, for example after a cutting-out session. Just drop the trimmings in the carrier bag.)

- A pencil on a string, tied to the bed head, may prevent a crisis.
- If a toy with many small pieces is top favourite, try putting a picture frame (without the glass, of course) on the table. It should keep everything like Lego bricks, or the tiny accessories for 'Play People' within bounds.

What to Do

- Activity books according to the ability of the child.
- Magic painting, (only requires a paintbrush and a little clear water to convert a boring grey picture into a blaze of colour!)
- Ordinary painting and tracing books, books of puzzles. These are a useful stand-by. Given a new painting book and a box of paints many a child has been tempted to fill in a little on every page, and then consider the job done. Sometimes, it is better to take out just one page for the child to fill in completely, and keep the rest of the book for another occasion.

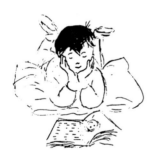

- Reading. When opportunity offers, raid the charity shops and car boot sales and have a little collection of books in reserve. When my children were poorly, my neighbour would arrive with some books from her children's selection for us to borrow. These were very welcome at the time, and I soon learnt to reciprocate if her children were confined to bed!
- Cutting out. For children who can safely be left with scissors, this activity will happily pass the minutes. Try offering an old mail-order catalogue. Perhaps cutting out the people to make paper dolls will be a starting point. Then how about planning a holiday for them, choosing the luggage and all the things to pack inside?

See also
Making a Scrapbook, p. 52.

- 'Silly pictures' are fun to make. Perhaps start with a glamorous kitchen, and add a horse drinking from the sink! The child's sense of humour will soon take over!

- How many things can you pack in a matchbox? This is a leftover idea from my days in the Brownies! It was great fun then, and still has an appeal for children with nimble fingers. It need only take seconds to prepare. Put any small item that comes to hand on a tray. Turn out that useful pot where all stray articles end up, and you may find a coin, a Smartie top, a paper clip, a tiny button or two, a key, a used stamp, a shoelace, a tiny toy ... need I go on? Challenge the child to fit in as many items as possible into the matchbox.

- Stacking Christmas Cards. Arrange the first card as though displaying it on the mantelpiece. Lay the second card horizontally across it. Repeat the process until the stack topples over!

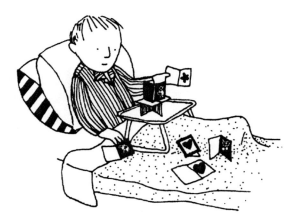

- Spot It. Give the child a list of things to spot, and tick off when successful. In hospital, this could be a nurse, Doctor, physiotherapist, thermometer, bowl of fruit, visitor, bandage, etc. At home, the window may provide a view of the street and the list might include a lorry, a red car, a lady with an umbrella, a baby in a pram, etc. Perhaps introduce a points system?

- Games for one. Solitaire with pegs or marbles. Card games of Patience. Pencil games like word search or crosswords for children.
- Tapes, videos and computers.

See also
Jigsaws, p. 47.
Many crafts , hobbies and art activities, pp. 75–83.
Toys to Make—the Instant and Quick sections, p. 115.

Play for two or more

BABY PLAY

Tickling games

What parent can resist blowing a 'raspberry' on a baby's tummy and being rewarded with his chuckle of delight! A traditional tickling game is called 'Round and Round the Garden'. Hold the baby's hand, palm upwards, in yours.

Say slowly:

Round and round the garden, like a teddy bear,
(draw circles on the palm of his hand in time to
   the words),
One step, Two step,
(walk your fingers up his arm)
And TICKLE me under there!
(tickle the baby under his chin or any other
   suitable place!).

It is easy to make up little games like this on the spot. When I changed my baby's nappy, he loved the feeling of freedom and would wave his legs about. We evolved a simple routine that never failed to please. I would cradle his heels in my hands and with a cycling movement we would go 'Slowly, slowly ... up the hill ... and down the other side' in double quick time! This had to be repeated over and over, and certainly helped to make nappy changing a fun time!

To and Fro

This is probably the first game a baby learns to play. You give him a toy, he hands it back to you. You are pleased and smiles are exchanged before you offer it to him again. He likes your reaction, so hands it back! And so the game proceeds. When the baby can sit securely, he may be ready for the simplest of all ball games. Just aim for his hand and slowly roll a large and colourful ball across the floor towards it. When he 'catches' the ball, he will probably want to put it in his mouth and generally explore it. After a while, he will be willing to give it up for the joy of having it bowled to him again. Some children like to sit with their legs apart, forming a sort of harbour. This certainly makes it easier for them to field the ball. The next stage is for him to try to return the ball to you. When he realises how difficult it is to aim straight, I guess his sense of humour will come to the fore and he will have more fun deliberately mis-aiming and making you chase after the ball!

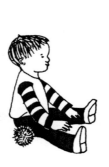
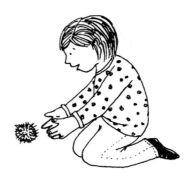

Peep-Bo

This is another old favourite. When you have the baby's attention, just hide your face behind your hands, open them and 'Bo!' It's the anticipated surprise that never seems to lose its appeal.

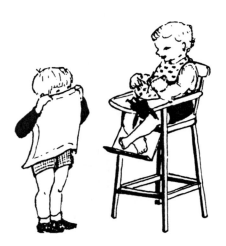

GAMES FOR THE NEXT STAGE

Match Me

Quick and Long-lasting

This is one of the simplest games I ever invented. Squares of coloured card are placed on the table. Objects matching those colours are stored in a bag. The game is to take these out one by one, and put them on the appropriate card. It makes an ideal introduction to other games, for it teaches the children to take turns and to watch how a game progresses.

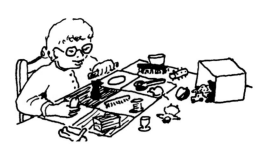

Materials
- Squares of card, using the primary colours and green or, for older children add more exotic colours like shocking pink, purple, rust, lavender, etc. (Remember you also have to supply objects in that colour!)
- Objects to match the colours on the cards, e.g. plastic clothes pegs, large buttons, reels of cotton, small toys (perhaps a red car, a blue cup and saucer, etc.), short lengths of ribbon, large beads ... There is room for ingenuity here. In my game, I have a white square and a shell, a plastic daisy, a tiny bottle brush and a piece of clear glass, now cloudy, that has been worn smooth by the sea. (All these pass for white.) On the brown square the children put a fir cone, a little wooden horse, a patch of fur fabric and a plastic pot, all coloured brown.
- A draw string bag for storing all the pieces.

Method
To play the game, the children sit round a table or in a group on the floor. An adult is in charge to name the colours and objects and, if necessary, keep control of the bag and make sure all the objects reach their correct destination. The coloured card squares are spread out. The children take it in turns to dip in the bag, pick out an object and place it on the correct square. There are no winners or losers. The game is over when all the objects have been matched to their squares.

Colour Dominoes

Quick

This home-made game of dominoes is suitable for children who cannot yet count or recognise the patterns of dots on the black and white commercial version. It is a simple colour matching game, which some children can make for themselves. Each card domino has two different coloured circles on its face. The game is to place the dominoes end-to-end so that the circle on the right side of one matches up to the circle on the left side of the following one, and so on all down the line.

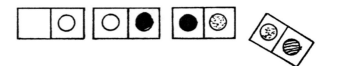

The summer holidays were approaching and one of the toy library members was heading for a caravan holiday. The weather forecast was not promising, so Mum made a hasty visit to the toy library to stock up on wet weather activities that might come in handy in a restricted space. On the 'Help Yourself' table were some kits for making a set of colour dominoes. I had invented this simple version of the game when my own children were little and it came in handy again in this situation. Each kit consisted of plenty of card rectangles and several sheets of large, circular, white Blick labels, which are sold at most stationers. The children could colour the circles with felt pens, only two of each colour, peel them off the backing paper and stick them carefully to the card rectangles. The easiest way of making sure the colours will match correctly (and the game will work) is to lay the card rectangles out in a row, like the carriages in a train. Leave the left half of the first one blank and stick a red circle to the right half. Stick the other red circle to the left half of the second rectangle, and a new colour to the right half. Its pair goes on the next rectangle, and so on all along the line, ending with a blank.

Lotto games

Lotto games for the young consist of two sets of pictures. One set is printed on the baseboards and the other set on individual cards which, in play, are matched to the baseboards. Usually all the small cards are muddled up and placed face downward in the middle of the table. Each child has a baseboard and takes it in turn to take a picture from the central pool. If it matches a picture on her baseboard she keeps it, if not, it is returned to the pool and the child waits for her turn to come round again. It takes quite a long time to play the game this way. For young children or those with a short attention span, I change the rules a little! Everyone has a baseboard, but the method of distributing the matching cards can vary according to the needs of the players. The leader turns up the first card and says the name of the object on it. The one who needs it for her baseboard claims it and puts it on top of its matching picture. If nobody recognises the word, she shows the picture to the children. The game continues until all the baseboards are covered. If played competitively, the first baseboard to be covered is the winner – BINGO!

A First Lotto

Long-lasting

Bought lotto games may not be suitable for young children. The pictures are often too complicated, the pieces too numerous, and the time taken to finish the game too long. The solution to all these problems is to make your own ... a tailor-made version.

This simple adaptation of the game is really just picture matching made into a group activity for, say, four players. It helps children understand the idea of matching a picture to a baseboard. In this case the matching picture is put beside the one on the baseboard and not on top of it. Now it is patently clear when the pictures are matched correctly. The eyes of every child will be following the matching process to make sure each player gets it right!

Materials
- Cardboard for the number of baseboards required, and for the matching cards. (I used the fronts and backs of soap powder packets for my first set.)
- Pairs of pictures. Picture Identification labels from an Educational Supplier (p. 184) save a lot of trouble and make a professional looking job. Otherwise, gift wrapping paper may be suitable, or perhaps you can draw your own.
- PVA adhesive.
- Clear, sticky-backed plastic from a large stationers or Educational Suppliers.
- A container for all the pieces.

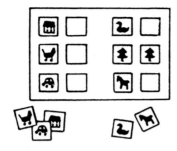

Method

You will need a quantity of pictures, for no pair must be used more than once. If you are drawing your own, you can increase the stock by making balloons in different colours, say blue on one pair of cards and red on another or draw one banana on one pair and two on another. The dimensions of the baseboard will depend on the number of pictures you use, plus enough space for blank squares beside each picture. Look at the illustration and rule pairs of squares in columns on your baseboard, leaving a gap between each pair of columns. Stick one picture from each pair onto the baseboard. Stick the other onto a small card. In play, this will be placed beside its partner on the baseboard. Wait until the adhesive is thoroughly dry, then cover all the pieces with sticky-backed plastic.

Lottos do not necessarily have to be pictorial. The game works just as well if you substitute colours, textures, shapes, patterns, or numbers.

Leafy Lotto

Long-lasting

This lotto is beautiful to look at and has a certain novelty value. It is made from real pressed leaves. Ideally, the children help to collect them, two of each shape, as nearly identical as possible. Press the leaves flat, between pages of blotting paper or newsprint and place them under a pile of books. Leave for about ten days, until the leaves have dried out and are really flat. Select the best pairs. Use one from each to mount on a baseboard and the other for the matching small card. A tiny dab of adhesive on each leaf is sufficient to anchor it in place. All the cards must be protected with clear sticky-backed plastic.

Other board games

A child who has learnt to play matching games, like the ones above, is ready to move onto board games where the moves are governed by the throwing of a dice. This is quite a large step for some young children to make. Take for example the game of 'Snakes and Ladders'. One of the major problems

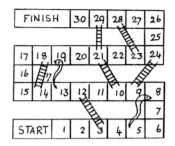

with the commercial version is that the children cannot always remember in which direction they should be travelling. They have been encouraged to move from left to right (the way we read and write) and suddenly they are asked to go the opposite way. Moreover, they must now start at the bottom and work their way to the top! All this is particularly confusing, if the child is not sure of the higher numbers, for the commercial version has 100 squares. As a preparation for the commercial game, I have made a simplified version as illustrated. The child must still move his counter in alternate directions, but the gap between the lines makes it much easier to follow the route. My simplified version also meanders from the bottom to the top of the board, but it has only 30 squares. It has more ladders than snakes so that the game does not last too long!

For beginners, I use a dice with only one, two and three spots. Each appears twice and the opposite sides always add up to four. It is easy to make a dice from a small wooden cube brick. Make the spots with felt pen or glue on tiny paper circles. (If the weight of the brick is a problem, make a small plastic one as described on p. 152).

COPY CAT GAMES

These seem to have a universal child appeal. 'Follow my leader' can be a winner for children in wheelchairs, motorised or not, especially if played out of doors and a slight element of surprise can be introduced, such as passing under a low tree, going down a small slope or manoeuvring between obstacles on the lawn.

Here are some more old favourites:

Simon Says

Simon (the leader) is very bossy. If Simon says an order, the players must instantly obey. If the action is not prefaced by 'Simon says', the players must ignore it. The game is usually played with thumbs only but, of course, it can be adapted to the mobility of the group. The leader might say: 'Simon says thumbs up'; (everyone obeys instantly). 'Thumbs down'; (everyone remains with their thumbs up, because Simon has not told them to do otherwise!). 'Simon says suck one thumb'; (The children obey, leaving one thumb still up). And so the game progresses. It is best played at speed, so that the children must really listen to the commands. These might include: twiddle your thumbs, thumbs down, thumbs sideways, clap your thumbs together, put your thumbs on your ears ... and so on.

Do This, Do That

This is really a variation on 'Simon Says', except that any body movement can be used. 'Do This' is the order and the children must copy the action— perhaps put their hands on their shoulders. 'Do That' and they must ignore the command.

Odd Bods

This is another imitation game, but this time the actions are cumulative. The first player says 'I saw an odd bod scratching his ear'. Everyone does the action. The second player says: 'I saw an odd bod scratching his ear and blinking his eyes'. Everyone adds blinking to ear scratching. The third player might add 'hunching his shoulders' or 'putting his tongue out', (very popular this, because it is RUDE!). The game usually has to come to an early end, because the players can't play for laughing!

VERBAL GAMES

The King of the Castle lost his Hat

This is an observation game similar to 'I Spy with My Little Eye'. It is suitable for young children who know the names of some colours, but are not yet too sure of letters and their sounds. Each turn is prefaced by the nonsense rhyme:

The King of the Castle lost his hat,
Some say this and some say that,
But I SAY (said with great emphasis!) Mr Red.

Everyone must look around the room for a red object, name it, and hope that they have picked the right one. The successful child has the next turn, says the rhyme and names the colour of another object. The game can be made slightly more complicated by naming two colours and choosing smaller objects. For instance 'black and silver' might be the knob on the television.

I Spy

Just in case you missed out on this traditional game, here is how to play it. The first player says: 'I spy with my little eye something beginning with ... B'. All the players then try to guess the object in the room beginning with that letter. The one who guesses correctly has the next turn. If this turns out to be nearly always the same child, vary the rules, so that everyone can have a turn in rotation.

**The Parson's Cat,
The Minister's Cat,
The Neighbour's Cat**

This game has many names, but they all amount to the same thing. It is an alphabet game and each player in turn has to think of an adjective to describe the unfortunate cat! The game might progress like this:

> *The Parson's cat is an Aggressive cat.*
> *The Parson's cat is a Beautiful cat.*
> *The Parson's cat is a Cautious cat.*
> *The Parson's cat is a Delightful/Dangerous/*
> *Dainty* (take your pick!) *cat*, and so on all
> through the alphabet.

I Went Shopping

This is a memory game. Each player must remember what previous players have bought and adds another item to the shopping list. The first player says: 'I went shopping and I bought ... a bag of potatoes.' The second player says: 'I went shopping and I bought a bag of potatoes and a tube of tooth paste'. And so on, until the list becomes too long for anyone to remember.

Variations on the game are 'I went on holiday and I took ...' or 'I packed a parcel and put in it ...'

**Hungry Harry
(or Harriet)**

This is yet another memory game. It can either be played soberly and the items mentioned perhaps alphabetically, or it can be farcical with Hungry

Harry's appetite becoming more and more ridiculous. (This is usually the most popular version!) Hungry Harry says: 'I feel so hungry I could ... eat an apple'. The next Hungry Harry eats an apple and a banana, and so on, perhaps including in the diet an elephant or a sack of potatoes, or whatever absurd item comes to mind. Of course, the gourmet's name can be altered to meet the occasion. (Hungry Harriet perhaps?)

Kim's Game

This is a game needing both observation and memory skills. It is not as verbal as the ones above, but it can lead to plenty of conversation, if the items in the game are chosen with that in mind. It is quick and easy to set up and can be adapted to fit most situations. Basically a collection of objects is placed on a tray. These might include a key, a button, a rubber band, a small toy, a picture postcard of a far away place, an object the children have never seen before ... Whatever comes to hand. The children all look at the collection carefully and try to memorise the positions of all the objects. They turn away and one item is removed. They look again and must try to name the missing item. It is then replaced. As the children become familiar with the contents of the tray, more objects can gradually be added to make the memory task more difficult. The children could now name the new item.

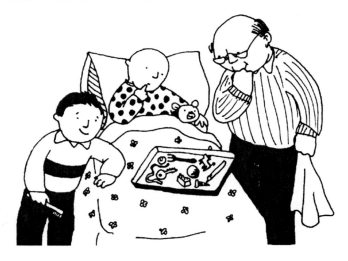

Play this game on the beach, and a circle drawn in the sand can represent the tray. Inside the circle could be stones, shells, scraps of seaweed, lolly sticks, etc. Play it in the park with twigs, leaves and pebbles.

PENCIL AND PAPER GAMES

The Dotty Game

Everyone has a small sheet of paper and makes five prominent dots at random. The paper is passed on to his neighbour, who must try to draw a picture or the outline of an object, joining up all the dots in the process.

Head, Body and Legs

This is an old favourite that can be played by children who are not yet capable writers and spellers. The children sit in a circle and all are given a strip of paper and a pencil. Everyone draws a head and neck at the top of the paper, then turns the top down firmly so that the head is hidden, but the two lines for the neck are still showing. All the papers are passed round to the next player who keeps the head hidden and draws the body—attached to the lines for the neck—leaving four short lines to indicate where the legs must go. The paper is turned down again so that the body is hidden. The papers change hands and this time the legs and feet are added before the paper is turned down once more. On go the papers to the next player, who writes a name at the bottom of the strip. The papers change hands for the last time. If even the writing of the name is still beyond the children, this last stage could be omitted. The strips are unfolded to reveal the (hilarious?) portrait. Everyone shares the jokes.

Consequences

This is a popular pencil and paper game for older children. It is also played on a strip of paper and is similar to the one above. Everyone begins by writing a boy's name. The paper is turned down and passed on to the next player who writes 'met', followed by a girl's name. More folding of paper and passing on. The game continues with 'At' ..., 'He said to her' ...,

'She said to him' ..., And the consequence was ... After the final passing on, everyone reads out their Consequence.

The Categories Game

Each player is given a sheet of paper and a pencil. In turn, one calls out a category such as: boy's name, girl's name, make of car, a river, a town, a country, a flower, a tree, a bird, an animal, etc., as many as possible. The players write these as a list down the left-hand side of the paper. Encourage small writing, then the paper can be used for several games. Next, a letter must be chosen. A novel way of doing this is for one child to choose the number of a page in a book (say one hundred and one). Another says which line of print (say the fifth) and a third names a number (say four) which means that the chosen letter for this game will be the fourth one in from the margin on line five of page one hundred and one! Now all the players must try to fill in their list with words beginning with the selected letter. If this turns out to be 'A' the list above might read 'Adam, Anne, Audi, Amazon, Amsterdam, Austria, etc. Everyone scores one point for a correct word. A player who thinks of a name that nobody else has written down scores two points. A new letter is chosen and the game can continue until there is no more room on the page.

The Word Game

Each player writes down the same long word, say 'Christmas'. The game is to write down as many short words as possible using only the letters in that word. Scoring can be as above, with an extra point for a word only one child has thought of, or points can be given for longer words. Come to an agreement on the rules before you start!

Boxes

This is a game for two players. It begins with a neat page of dots arranged in lines and columns—say ten by ten. The players take turns to join up a pair of dots. The object of the game is to make the final stroke to complete a box. A player who succeeds in this can put his initial in it. At first the action is slow and it is easy to draw a line that will not allow

100

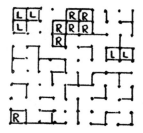

the opponent to make a box, but as the number of lines increases this becomes much more difficult. When all the dots are joined up at the end of the game, the player with the most initials in the boxes is the winner.

Hangman

This is a gruesome game that is popular with good spellers. It is a game for two. The first player 'A' thinks of a long word, and on a sheet of paper indicates each letter with a dash. The second player 'B' guesses a letter. If it appears in the word, 'A' writes it over the correct dash. If it is not in the word, 'A' starts to draw a hangman's noose. For every wrong guess another part is added. First the upright post, then the horizontal beam, the rope, the noose, the player's head, body, arms, legs. Hopefully 'B' has guessed all the letters in the word long before he meets his doom! The players change roles and 'B' challenges 'A' to guess his word before he may be hanged.

SOME LIGHT-HEARTED LIFESAVERS

The whole of this book is concerned with fun, but this little section is all about silly fun! Everything on the list can be set up in minutes, if not seconds, and all the activities have proved to be winners with my own children and many more besides. Some items— like making orange peel teeth—have been around for many years but, in the busy lives of the present day, it is easy to forget about such simple pleasures. A quick flip through the following pages may remind you of your own childhood and, perhaps, you can add your own 'silly fun' to the list.

Blowing a Mound of Bubbles

An economical recipe for bubble mixture is on p. 177.

Children often discover for themselves how to make a mound of bubbles when they blow vigorously through a straw into their beaker of

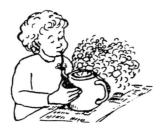

milk—and are probably scolded for their bad manners! Given some bubble mixture in a pudding basin and a drinking straw, a child can raise an impressive pile of bubbles in seconds. The little girl in the illustration is blowing down the spout of a teapot. You might try covering a pudding basin with a colander and watching the bubbles appear through the holes. To blow a smaller mound, try the bubble blower below.

A Special Bubble Blower

Quick

Jo Sweeney,
Hospital Play Specialist

Jo visited a Science Workshop in the USA where she watched children raising mounds of bubbles by this simple and economical method. Each child was given a yoghurt pot, a circle of terry towelling to fit over the top and a rubber band to keep it in place. A small hole had been punched fairly near the top of the yoghurt pot and a drinking straw was inserted into this. Next, *only the terry towelling top* was dipped in the bubble mixture. Now the children could blow through their straws and create huge sausages of bubbles! This method is excellent for children in bed for there is no surplus bubble mixture to spill. It is also very hygienic for the drinking straws can be replaced, and the terry towelling top and yoghurt pot well washed.

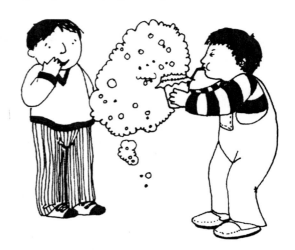

Blowing a Single Bubble

One bath night my children discovered that a cotton reel (floating around as a bath toy!) made a good bubble pipe. One end was gently wiped over the damp soap to form a membrane. A gentle stream of breath directed through the other end of the central hole produced a beautiful bubble!

The Ultimate in Bubble Blowing

I guess you have marvelled at a ship in a bottle, but how about a child in a bubble? Two Hospital Play Specialists demonstrated how this could be done. They spread bubble mixture over the surface of a large tray and made a loop of string large enough to encircle a child. They attached four string handles to the loop, at equal distances apart. They dipped the string circle into the bubble mixture, waited a few seconds for it to become impregnated. Then they carefully lifted the loop, keeping the membrane intact, held it high above the child, then smartly lowered it, trapping him inside the bubble!

Hocus Pocus

Instant

A Swiss Paediatric Occupational Therapist taught me this wonderful game and I suspect she invented it. It can be played by a small group of children mature enough to be able to take turns. It has the perfect formula—a ritual sentence, eating sweets, and everyone is a winner! It only requires a small plate, a spoon and a supply of small edible items—say sweets, but of course small pieces of fruit, or different breakfast cereals would do just as well. Imagine a small bunch of children gathered round a leader. One child is chosen to hide her eyes. The leader puts three edible items on the plate—say an orange, a yellow and a red sweet. Everyone chants

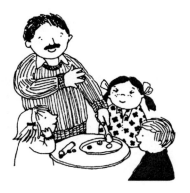

'Hocus Pocus, don't eat ME' and the leader points to one of the sweets, say the red one, putting a spell on it. The chosen child uncovers her eyes and picks up a sweet. If she chooses the red one first (with the spell on it) she can eat that one but no more. If she starts with one of the others she is in luck, for there is no spell on them. So whatever her choice, she is certain to eat one sweet, and she might possibly have all three.

The children watching soon become involved in the game, clapping when a child makes a lucky guess and groaning when the sweet with the spell on it is chosen. At the end of the game, share out the remaining sweets.

Gloop

Almost Instant

This strange mixture is made by mixing together a packet of cornflour and enough water (about a cup full) to turn it into a fairly stiff paste. This has a fascinating feel. Pour the mixture onto a Formica-topped table or tray, and it will have a strange amoeba-like will of its own. Pile it into a peak and it will subside into a puddle. Push one side and it will bulge out elsewhere. Dribble it through your fingers and weird shapes are formed. The mixture can be stored for a short while in a screw-topped jar. If it thickens up, just add a little more water.

Making Silly Pictures

Quick

This activity requires plenty of old magazines, mail-order catalogues, old Christmas cards etc., some plain paper for the background, scissors and paste. Pritt Stick is ideal for children in bed providing you can persuade them to replace the cap between uses. Otherwise it soon dries out.

As the heading suggests, the aim of the artist is to create as silly a picture as possible—perhaps a horse in the kitchen or a boat perched on top of the Church spire. Then the pictures are passed round for everyone to spot the deliberate mistake and share the joke.

Compiling a Book of Riddles and Jokes

Quick

This can be a time-filling fun activity for a group of literate children. Provide everyone with a little book made from an old Christmas Card with a few blank pages tied inside, and a pencil. Set a time limit. Everyone fills his book with his favourite jokes and, at the end of the time, turns are taken to read them all out. If this goes down like a lead balloon, because the children declare they do not know any jokes, let them research their comics or remind each other of some they have heard on Children's TV.

Wax Resistant Messages

Quick

For this you will need some stubs of cheap white candle, a quantity of scrap paper, some watery paint and a fat paint brush. Write a message on the scrap paper with the stub of the candle. (Press quite hard.) Deliver the message to a friend. He must cover the paper with a wash of watery paint to reveal the waxy message.

Ghost Pictures or Butterflies

Quick

Both of these activities require plenty of scrap paper, some fairly sloppy powder paint and a paintbrush. To make a ghost, fold a piece of paper in half and paint your name large, in joined-up writing, along the fold. Refold the paper and press along the crease to smear the paint. Open out the paper to see the shape of your 'ghost'.

A butterfly is made in the same way. Working quite quickly (before the paint dries) paint in half the head and body of the butterfly along the crease in the paper. Add one of its wings. Fold up the paper again and press the top of the sheet to the bottom. Open out the page to see the whole butterfly revealed.

Orange Peel Teeth

Instant

Next time you eat an orange, remove the peel in as large pieces as possible. Carve out two strips to be your top and bottom sets. Nick each strip to indicate teeth. Tuck your new set behind your lips and look in the mirror!

Bringing the world to the child

Children who have restricted mobility and limited energy are obviously not able to explore the world around them as easily as their more energetic friends. They are likely to welcome an adult or child who has the time and imagination to bring the world (or part of it!) to them. This may seem an easy task but, in practice, it can often be difficult to come up with ideas. One simple suggestion is to look outside the window and bring inside a sample of what is out there. In spring, this might just mean gathering a bunch of twigs from the garden. Pop them in a vase, or better still let the child arrange them, and in a very short time they will gradually unfold their leaves—or blossoms if you include some prunings from the fruit trees!

GROWING THINGS

Here are some popular ideas for easy indoor gardening. If your child has not already tried them and you think they might appeal, give them a chance. They have interested hoards of children in their time!

Mustard or cress

Mustard grows slightly faster, but has a hot taste. If the product is going to be eaten, cress may be more palatable. Either of these seeds can be grown on a circle of damp blotting paper or cotton wool on a saucer, but it is more fun to grow them as part of the creatures described below.

A Hairy Humpty Dumpty

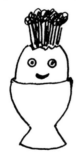

Eat a boiled egg, and save the shell. Wash it carefully and stuff it lightly with cotton wool. Put the shell in an eggcup (for easy handling) and with felt pens, give it a face. Moisten the cotton wool and sprinkle on the seeds. Make sure they never dry out and, in a very short time (say two days), little roots, will start to sprout. By about the end of the week, Humpty should be due for a haircut!

A Cress Hedgehog

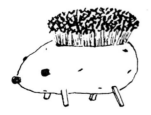

For this you need a small potato, and four matchsticks for the legs. With a teaspoon, scoop out a hollow in the potato—where you want the 'spines' to grow. Break the heads off the matches and use two for the eyes. (Dispose of the other two safely.) Press the rest of the matchsticks into the potato at appropriate places to represent the legs. Fill the hollow in the back with cotton wool, moisten it and sprinkle it with seeds as above.

Leaves from the tops of vegetables

The tops of root vegetables will sprout fresh leaves if kept damp and never allowed to dry out. Try carrots, parsnips, beetroot, swedes or turnips. Slice about $2\frac{1}{2}$ cm (1") from the top of the vegetable and place it in a saucer with a little water in it. New leaves should start to shoot within a day or two. The top of a pineapple will sprout like a miniature palm tree if given the chance. Cut off the top 5 cm (2") and leave to dry off for about a week. Then plant it in a pot of sandy soil and keep it moist. It should start to sprout in about a month.

Mung beans

Mung beans bought from a Health Food Shop will soon develop into bean sprouts. Soak them in cold water for about four hours, then spread them on a tray covered with damp blotting paper. To produce the whitest shoots, it is best to cover them with black polythene, but then of course the child cannot watch them grow. Forget this if you are not aiming at speedy growth and don't mind if your shoots are not so white. When the crop is ready, wash it and eat it.

Hyacinths or onions

In the autumn it is possible to buy a special glass (at garden centres etc.) for growing a hyacinth in water. The glass is quite tall and widens out into a dish shape on the top to receive the bulb. The glass is filled with water until the base of the bulb is just touching it. Then all you have to do is make sure the water level does not drop, and wait for the roots to reach down into the water. Ultimately, the flower will appear.

Growing an onion does not need a special glass. Just find a jam jar and four cocktail sticks. Poke the cocktail sticks into the base of the onion so that it will sit across the top of the jam jar with its end just below the rim. Fill the jam jar with water and await results! With luck you should grow a healthy crop of leaves and even a flower.

MAKING A MINIATURE GARDEN

I know a little girl who will happily spend an afternoon making an outdoor garden for the pixies. She finds a tree with gnarled roots, to make the walls. She lines the space between the roots with moss gathered from here and there, and then lays out her garden. Small stones make the paths, wild flowers 'grow' in the moss and small leafy twigs represent the trees. Sometimes the pixies even have a twig house—and a tea set made from acorn cups set out on a leafy tablecloth.

This kind of outdoor play may not be possible for some children, but creating a tiny garden in a container is always an option. The easiest miniature garden can be made in a saucer. Just fill it with damp moss and poke in small short-stemmed flowers and leaves.

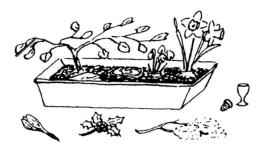

For more elaborate horticulture use a meat tin filled with soil. Tiny plants, kept moist, will last for quite a long time. Lawns can be made from moss, paths from sand, gravel or tiny stones, and a pond from a handbag mirror. Adding blossoms to the garden can be a problem, as the plants will probably grow to bush size before they flower. One way round this is to sink small containers—such as thimbles, potted meat jars or cut-down film cartons—into the soil, and fill them with tiny blossoms. I introduced this idea to my young toy library friend, Gavin. Before long his imagination was at work. He made a fence from lolly sticks, and took the ducks from his farmyard to swim on the pond. Convincing bulrushes, made from cocktail sticks with a blob of brown Plasticine on the top, grew round the edge. People and seats for them to rest on (while they admired the garden?) were fashioned from more Plasticine.

MAKING A WORMERY

Children with a scientific turn of mind may like to watch a wormery in action. This can be quite easy to make. All you need is a large plastic kitchen storage jar (or an empty sweet jar begged from the corner shop). Fill it with alternate layers of soil and sand (not too dry) dig up a few worms, and sprinkle some dry leaves on the top. In time, the worms will drag the leaves into the jar and the layers of soil and sand will be mixed together. Worms come nearer to the surface of the soil in wet weather, so make sure the contents of the jar do not dry out by giving the soil a light shower now and then. Don't forget to return the worms to the garden when they have served their purpose.

WEATHER WATCHING

Don't rely on the weatherman to do the forecast. Help the child to observe, and keep a record, of the daily happenings. Point out cloud formations and see what kind of weather they predict, and perhaps make a note of the hours of sunshine. At a less scientific level, I remember my children watching the raindrops on the windowpane and having races with them!

Making a weather chart will fill in a few moments of each day. This can be just a sheet of paper with a square for every day and symbols or pictures drawn in. However, it can be made more interesting if an element of collage is included in the pictures, e.g. dabs of cotton wool stuck on to represent white fluffy clouds, grey paper clouds for rainy days—with the rain drawn falling out of them—a tree covered with tracing paper to symbolise fog ... and so on.

For children who are unable to draw, a member of the family can perhaps make a simple weather chart from a circle of card about the size of a dinner plate, with a pointer attached to the centre. (Use a paper clip—the kind with legs that splay out.) Supposing sunny, windy, rainy, cloudy, foggy and snowy are chosen as the types of weather that can be illustrated easily. Divide the card circle into six segments like the slices of a pie, and draw a weather picture or symbol in each. Fix the pointer to the centre of the circle, and all the child has to do is position it to point at the right segment for the weather of the day.

A Weather Doll

At the time, I wanted a simple and unusual weather indicator for a small child with a visual impairment. In this situation, pictures and symbols were useless, so I tried a three-D approach. The result pleased the child in question and, when it eventually found its way to the toy library shelves, many other (sighted) children also liked to play with it. I began with a paper doll from a cheap cut-out book. This gave me a figure and a wardrobe of paper clothes for her to wear. These were too flimsy for my purpose, so I used them as inspiration for a cloth equivalent before they found their way to the wastepaper basket. The figure was mounted on plywood and its outline cut out with a jigsaw. It was inserted into a slot in a firm wooden block, so that it would stand erect and not be easily knocked over. The clothes were what I considered suitable for basic types of weather! It took me a while to work out how to dress such a stiff and unbending doll. Hats were easy. They just perched on her head. Ponchos were just a square of woolly fabric with a slit in the centre for the doll's head to slip through. Skirts and sundresses wrapped round her body with the back seam closed with a Velcro fastening. Other body clothes slotted over the doll's head and hung down fore and aft like a sandwich board! Small strips of Velcro at the side seams made for a better fit.

The outfits included sundresses with shady hats to match, and on rainy days the doll could wear a plastic cape and sou'wester. When the weather turned chilly, our doll was decked out in a warm poncho, a long scarf to keep her neck cosy and a woolly bobble hat to complete the outfit. All the clothes were kept neatly folded in a little doll's suitcase that greatly added to the attraction of the activity.

See also
A Weather mobile, p. 22.

STAMP COLLECTING

This absorbing hobby (for some) has already been mentioned briefly in the alphabetical list of crafts and hobbies, *see* p. 82. As a way of bringing the world to the child, it is full of potential. Collections grow by swapping and this can lead to unexpected friendships. The stamps themselves are full of interest and often illustrate the wild life, scenery or famous people connected to the country.

For young children, stamp collecting need not be the serious business it can become for enthusiastic adult philatelists. The story of six-year-old Nigel illustrates this rather well. He belonged to the toy library several years ago. His condition confined him to a wheelchair, but his mind was always racing ahead of the restraints that his body imposed on him. One day I took in a few stamps from overseas, and Nigel's Mum pounced on them. On her way home, she bought a lever-arch folder, a pad of A4 paper and a Pritt Stick. This modest outlay led to an absorbing hobby for Nigel. He learnt to float the envelope backs off the stamps, wait for them to dry out, and then mount them on the A4 sheets in his impressive folder. Word soon spread around the members of the toy library and his

Dad's office. Before long he was receiving as many stamps as he could cope with. If one from a new country turned up, he would write the name of the country at the top of a clean page and insert it, alphabetically, in its rightful place in his folder. At his young age, there was no need to arrange his collection according to sets. He found enjoyment and satisfaction in just mounting the stamps on their correct page and gradually building up a sizeable collection. He was fascinated by the pictures on the stamps and wanted to know all about them. This was quite a strain on his parents! I guess that with modern computer technology, he could have discovered much interesting information for himself. He is now an adult, and I heard recently that he is heavily into 'proper' philately, and often consulted about rare specimens by his friends.

For more information, contact The British Philatelic Trust. This is an educational charity set up by the Post Office in 1981 to support philately. It produces a Stamps Fact Sheet which gives sources of supply, and recommends books, publications, exhibitions and places to visit. There is a UK Philately Website:www.ukphilately.org.uk.

For young collectors there is The Royal Mail Collectors Club, Freepost, NEA1431, Dept. 2397, Sunderland SR9 9XN. The Club runs a bi-monthly magazine with special offers, lists of pen pals etc. At the time of writing a two-year subscription costs £5.

See also
ABC of Crafts and Activities, for:
Birdwatching, p. 75.
Collections, p. 76.
Letter writing, p. 78

More quick and easy toys to make

The toys in this section are graded for difficulty. Those at the beginning are *Instant* or *Quick* and can probably be made by the children. Alternatively, an adult who is searching for a little novelty to take to a child in hospital or as a 'morale-raiser' at home might make them in a jiffy. They also come in handy as a little present for one child to make for another. Balls, dolls and puppets are grouped together, again with the *quick* and easy ones first.

The latter part of the chapter describes some *Long-lasting* toys I have made for a special child. Other adults might like to read about these and consider making something similar as an unusual present.

A SELECTION OF SMALL TOYS

A Helicopter

Instant

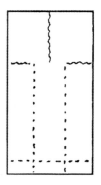

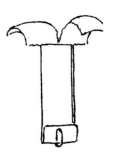

If your child is already a confident paper tearer he can have a go at this. All you need is a strip of paper, not too thick and heavy, about 8 × 20 cm (3 × 8″). A sheet of A4 paper folded from top to bottom and then again and cut into strips will make four helicopters.

Hold the paper horizontally and about 1/3 of the way along the top tear in about 1/3 of the way (consult the diagram). Fold in the long flap. Repeat the process with the other side and fold in the flap. You should now have a shape similar to a spade or a rectangular lollipop! Turn up the bottom of the central folded part. Carefully tear from the centre of the 'lollipop' to the folded part. You have now made the rotor blades! Bend one rotor blade away from you and the other towards you. Give them a slight curve as in the illustration. (Put your thumb under a blade and two fingers on top and gently squeeze.)

Now for the maiden flight! Hold the helicopter up high and just let go. (Do not throw it.) It should gently spiral its way to the floor, in the manner of a sycamore seed.

A Convection Snake

Very Quick

This is an almost instant toy that can be made by anyone who can confidently use scissors. Make several, and they can hang as part of a mobile. Make just one and balance the head on a pencil held in a cotton reel. Place it on a shelf over a radiator and the snake should slowly revolve in the upward warm air current.

Materials
- A circle of cartridge paper or thin card, about the size of a tea plate.
- Scissors.
- Felt pens.

Method

Start at the outside edge and slowly cut out a spiral that gets wider as you near the middle—like a real coiled-up snake. End with a blob for the head in the centre. Decorate the snake, both sides. Hang it from a string or rest it on a pencil as suggested above.

Lolly Stick Puzzles

Quick

Imagine four lolly sticks placed tidily edge-to-edge so that they make the shape of a raft. With a felt pen, the child writes her name across the centre two and decorates the edges with a pattern. Now muddle up the lolly sticks and try to return them to their original positions. This is the puzzle in its simplest form. Add more rows of lolly sticks and the child's surname can be added. Be even more ambitious and, with further rows of lolly sticks, the child's address might be included too!

Alternatively, substitute a picture for the writing or make a simple pattern. Diagonal lines ruled across the lolly sticks and then coloured in as stripes can make a challenging puzzle. Before the lolly sticks are decorated, hold them temporarily in position with strips of masking tape.

The children will probably think of other ways of arranging the lolly sticks, perhaps vertically, like a fence, instead of horizontally, or slightly overlapping each other like steps. There is plenty of scope for originality here.

A Button Tapper

Quick

Robert Race,
Maker of Automata
and Adult Toys

I learnt to make this delightful little toy when attending one of Robert's toy-making courses. I believe the idea came originally from India. It can be made in seconds and has great novelty value. It makes an excellent 'Doodle toy'. Its life is not infinite, so that by the time the noise it makes starts to get on your nerves, the rubber band may break, and it is up to you whether or not you find another!

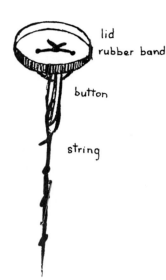

lid

rubber band

button

string

Materials

- A plastic lid for the top of the toy, perhaps from a plastic milk bottle or from a jar of Marmite, Bovril, etc.
- An elastic band.
- A coat button with holes large enough to accept the (cut) elastic band.
- A length of string—say a bit less than a metre—and thin enough to go through a hole in the button.

Method

Make two holes in the lid with an awl or other spiked tool. Cut the band and thread it through a hole in the button. Hold the lid upside down. Thread the loose ends of the band up through the two holes in the lid. Tie the ends together firmly, making sure the rim of the button is pulled quite tightly against the lid. Make knots at regular intervals all along the string. Thread one end through the button (the opposite hole to the one with the band through it) and tie it on firmly.

Now to make it work. Hold the lid with one hand and with the other gently pinch the string. As you slide your thumb and finger down the string, every time you reach a knot the button will pull away from the lid. As you pass the knot, the button will snap back against it. Perform this sliding action speedily, and you will make the sound of a heavy shower on a tin roof or a woodpecker at work! Do it more slowly, and you can imagine a clock ticking. I guess you will find this quite soothing and therapeutic. Be unselfish and now let your child have a go!

A Miniature Pop-up Dolly

Quick

This little novelty is a winner with children. At the toy library we keep a few in stock for emergencies! They come in handy as a tiny gift for a birthday child or to welcome a new member. One has even been known to distract a child in the middle of a temper tantrum and stop a rumpus!

Materials

- A lolly stick.

119

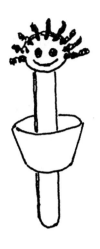

- Two tiny plastic milk cartons from a Motorway Services café, etc.
- A small circle of card for the face.
- Possibly some wool for hair, etc.

Method

Put one milk carton inside another for added strength. Cut a slot across the bottom, the width of the lolly stick (a job for an adult). Cut out a small circle of card for the head. Check that it will fit in the milk cartons. Draw a face on it, and perhaps give it hair or a hat? Glue it to one end of the lolly stick and insert the other in the milk cartons. Now you have a miniature pop-up dolly that can hide away and be made to pop up suddenly to give Grandma a surprise!

A Tunnel Pop-up Toy

Quick

Marianne
Willemsen-van Witsen

A ping-pong ball is partly hidden inside a tube as shown in the illustration. Push it down a little further, and a sharp pull on the ribbon will shoot it out of the tube—to be chased all over the floor by the energetic.

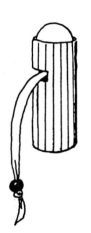

Materials

- A ping-pong ball.
- A cardboard tube (cut from the inside of a roll of paper towel.) Check that the ping-pong ball will fit easily inside it.
- Ribbon, about 2 1/2 cm (1″) wide and roughly four times the length of the tube.
- A bead for the end of the ribbon. This is optional, but it makes it easier to grasp.
- PVA adhesive.
- Decoration for the tube—paint, paper, Fablon or cloth.

Method

Cut a horizontal slit like a letterbox, fairly near the top of the cardboard tube. Make it just wide enough for the ribbon to slide through easily. Thread the ribbon through the slot to the inside of the tube. Pull it up and away from you, so that it comes out of the tube and over the edge. Stick it down the entire length of the 'back' of the tube. This will attach it firmly so that it will stand plenty of tugging. Thread the free end of the ribbon through the bead and tie a knot. Once the glue is dry, the toy is almost finished and ready for its trials. Push the ping-pong ball down inside the tube a little way. It will sit in the ribbon sling. Hold the tube in one hand and pull the ribbon smartly with the other. The ball will shoot out of the top. If you have a problem, it could be that the tube has become slightly squashed. Strengthen it with strips of paper—or find another one and start again! When you are satisfied the toy is working well, decorate the tube.

A Pop-up Matchbox

Quick

Marianne
Willemsen-van Witsen

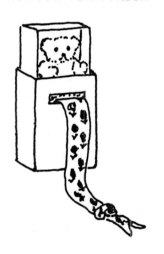

If you have already made the Tunnel Pop-up Toy, you will have no difficulty with this one. It works on the same principle, but the action is slower and less dramatic. Pull the ribbon, and the tray of the matchbox will rise most of the way out of its cover to reveal its hidden treasure!

Materials
- A matchbox.
- A short length of ribbon, say 20 cm (8″) long.
- A bead (optional).
- A decorative cover for the matchbox.
- Something to stick inside for the surprise—a tiny doll, a toy from a cracker, a face cut from a photograph?

Method
Remove the tray from the matchbox cover. Cut a slot in the cover, about 2 cm (3/4″) from the top, wide enough to take the ribbon. If you make the slot too near the top, the tray will come right out when the ribbon is pulled. If you make it too far down, the tray will not rise up properly. Even a simple little toy like this can have its technical hazards! Thread the ribbon through the slot to the inside of the box, then pull it up and over the back. Stick it along the entire length of the back. Insert the tray gently so that it sits in the ribbon sling, and press it down. The ribbon will

121

shorten as the tray disappears inside the cover. Tie a bead to the free end of the ribbon. Pull it gently to make sure the tray rises up as you expect. Take the tray out and decorate the part that will show. Then decorate the cover. The quickest way is to wrap it in coloured Sellotape. This will also cover the abrasive sides.

A Cup and Ball

Quick

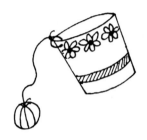

This traditional toy has given pleasure to children down the ages. It is pictured on an ancient Greek vase and we know that the little daughter of Marie Antoinette had one exquisitely carved in ivory called a bilboquet. It was a favourite in Victorian nurseries and, made in wood, it still turns up sometimes in gift shops and craft markets.

The toy is just a ball attached to a cup by a fairly long string. The aim is to swing the ball and catch it in the cup. This is not as easy as it might seem!

The ball should be fairly soft and light, so that if it flies into the child's face it will do no damage.

Materials
- For a woolly ball—see p. 124. To make one as illustrated here, you will need newspaper, kitchen foil and thin string or button thread.
- Thin string to attach the ball to the pot.
- A yoghurt pot, possibly covered with felt and trimming, or with strips of coloured paper stuck all over the outside. This will strengthen the yoghurt pot and has some cosmetic value.

Method
To make a newspaper ball, tightly crunch up half a sheet. Check that it will fit easily into the yoghurt pot. Wrap it in kitchen foil to give it some sparkle and glamour. Keep it in good shape by binding round it once with button thread or thin string and tie the ends together, but do not cut the thread. Continue binding tightly round the ball as if making lines of longitude on the globe! Tie the ends together again and add the attaching string. Make a small hole near the top of the yoghurt pot, poke the free end of the attaching string through it

and tie. Use a short string for beginners, and a longer one for the more confident.

Jumping Jacks

Quick

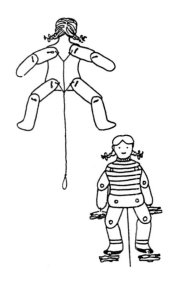

Jumping Jacks are traditional toys, usually made in wood. This version is in cardboard. The limbs are joined to the body with paper clips—the kind with 'legs' that open out—and are linked together with string. When the central string is pulled, the little figure will dance. In addition to joints at the shoulders and hips, the Jumping Jack illustrated has jointed knees and elbows. This makes for more exciting movement, but is not essential. Before you begin it is always sensible to make a paper pattern. You can experiment with the proportions of your Jumping Jack, and make sure it works well before going to the trouble of making the final toy.

Look at the illustration and work out the mechanics of making your Jack (or Jill) jump. Then draw the head and body in one piece. Make the neck fairly thick—for strength. Draw the arms and decide on their position. They must swivel on the paper fasteners, so as to be horizontal with the body when the connecting string is pulled fully down, and be almost hidden by the body when relaxed. Cut out the legs—longer than the arms and with suggested feet at the end. Paper clip them to the body and see how they look. When you are happy with your design, transfer your shapes to fairly thick cardboard and cut them out. Paint all the pieces. Fix the limbs in place with paper fasteners and string them together as shown in the illustration. For an added attraction, tie a string of foil milk bottle tops (with a button at the bottom of the string to stop them from sliding off) or a little bell to the hands and feet.

See also
Christmas Card Jigsaws, p. 49.
Making a Scrapbook, p. 52.
Colour Dominoes, p. 91.
A Special Bubble Blower, p. 102.

BALLS

When it comes to balls, a visit to the toy shop will provide you with plenty of choice, but you may be looking for one with sober habits that will not roll too fast. In this case the best idea is an evening of DIY! Here are some suggestions for slow moving balls:

A Woolly Ball

Easy, but time consuming

To make a ball about the size of a tennis ball, first cut two identical circles in card. The Cornflakes packet will do. Make the diameter about 10 cm (4″). Cut a hole in the centre of each, about 4 cm (1½″) wide. Hold the circles together and wind the wool over the edge and up through the centre, gradually working your way all round the ring. At this stage the ball resembles a ring doughnut. As the hole gradually fills up, you will need a needle threaded with wool to finish the winding. When you can hold the ring to your eye and cannot see through it, this part of the job is finished. Now take a pair of sharp-pointed scissors. At one point on the circumference of the circle, snip the wool until you come to the cardboard. Poke the scissors between the two circles of cardboard and continue to snip your way round the ring until all the wool has been cut. You now have lots of strands of wool sticking out each side of the cardboard circles. Ease the cardboard circles a little way apart. Using strong button thread TIGHTLY bind round the wool between the cardboard circles, finishing off with a sturdy knot. Snip the cardboard circles and pull them away. Fluff up the wool to make the ball a good shape and trim off any straggly ends.

Note
Making a ball like this can be an excellent way of using up odd ends of wool. Go for bright colours and include some dark ones to give contrast. Avoid too many pastel shades as the ball is likely to spend most of its life on the floor. Providing it is tightly tied together, the ball will wash well but it takes a long time to dry.

A Felt or Fabric Ball

Long-lasting

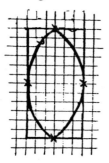

This ball is made in six petal-shaped segments like the one in the diagram. The length of each segment is three times its width, so it is easy to adjust the pattern to make a ball the size you want. If you need a strong ball, use a woven fabric. If it is likely to be soon outgrown, go for the easier option and use felt. This will not fray so the seams need not be oversewn, but it can wear thin, split or even have holes picked in it by busy little fingers, and, worst of all, it will not wash well. Its lovely bright colours and easiness to sew may perhaps outweigh all these disadvantages.

Materials

- Small piece of card for the template.
- Fabric—woven or felt.
- Polyester fibre for the stuffing.
- If you make the Popper Balls below, you will also need some Velcoins. These are the larger circles of Velcro easily obtained from a haberdashery department.

Method

Make a template the size you want, following the proportions in the illustration. Draw round it six times on the fabric. You can use the pencil lines as a stitching guide. Cut out the six segments. Pin them together and stitch up all the seams, leaving a little gap in the last one for inserting the stuffing. Turn the ball the right side out, stuff, and close the seam. If the segments at the 'North and South Poles' of the ball do not meet accurately, cover them up with a circle of felt!

Popper Balls

Long-lasting

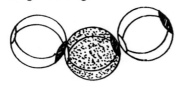

These are made exactly like the balls above, but are quite small, say 3 cm (1$\frac{1}{4}$") × 9 cm (3$\frac{3}{4}$"). When Velcoins are attached to the tops and bottoms, they can be joined together to make a necklace (quite safe, for if another child grabs it, it will simply fall apart). If you make the balls as identical pairs, they can come in useful for practising colour matching, counting in twos, etc.

Stuff each ball just firmly enough to give it a good shape. Do not overstuff or it may be too heavy to stick to its neighbour. Stitch the furry part of a Velcoin to each 'North Pole' and the rough half to the 'South Pole'.

A Patchwork Ball

Long-lasting

Betty Lewis,
Toy-maker for the
Kingston-upon-Thames
Toy Library

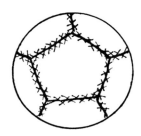

Betty makes beautiful patchwork balls with bells inside as presents for some of the babies and toddlers who come to the toy library. The balls are visually attractive, roll slowly, and the bell inside makes them even more desirable! Anyone already familiar with the technique of patchwork will have no difficulty in making one. The ball is made up of twelve five-sided patches. As these are sewn together, edge-to-edge mosaic fashion, they form the curved surface of the ball. Think of the multiple mirror facets of a disco ball reduced to a mere twelve shapes, and you will have a rough idea of the finished toy.

Materials
- Cardboard to make the template for the patches. Either trace off the one illustrated (diagram a) which will give you a ball of about 7 cm (3") diameter or, if you are good at geometry and want a larger one, scale it up (*see* diagram b).
- Fairly stiff paper for the patches.
- Small pieces of cotton or similar fabric. Choose the colours carefully to accentuate the mosaic nature of the ball.
- Embroidery thread (black looks good) for the herringbone stitch which covers the seams when the ball is stuffed.
- A plastic cat ball with a bell inside—from the pet shop.
- Polyester fibre.

a

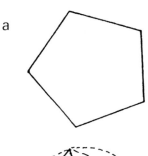

b

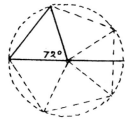

Method
Using the cardboard template, cut out (accurately!) twelve paper shapes. Before covering them with fabric, you may like to work out a colour scheme, or perhaps go for the easy option and just make every shape a different colour. As an experienced

patchworker, you will have your own ideas about this! Choose one shape to be the centre of the top of the ball. Working on the wrong side, oversew five shapes to it to form a dome—or a skull cap with a zigzag edge. Make a similar dome for the bottom of the ball. Still working on the wrong side, sew them together for most of the way round. Remove the paper backing to the shapes. Turn the ball the right side out, insert the cat ball and surround it with stuffing. Close the gap. As an optional extra, add to the strength and beauty of the ball by covering all the seams with herringbone stitch worked in three strands of embroidery thread.

DOLLS

This section is all about dolls that are quick and easy to make. (Some more than others!) Beautiful dolls abound in the shops, but to my mind there is nothing that can compare with a home-made one, stitched with care for a special child. Some of the dolls at the beginning of the chapter make excellent 'extras' if an imaginative game of playing 'Hospitals' or 'Schools' is the flavour of the day. Given a little help, the children may be able to make them for themselves, and perhaps even use them as dolls for their own dolls!

Instant Dolls

Loet Vos,
Museum of Childhood,
Toronto

Follow the drawings on the next page and within ten minutes you should end up with a rough and ready doll! Just the thing if you want plenty of people to add to a model, or extra inhabitants for the dolls' house. Children of about seven, with good hand function may be able to make these—perhaps with a little help in tying the knots. As you see, dressing them can be simplicity itself. As an added refinement, pipe cleaners can be rolled up in the cloth at stage one and will add a little stiffening to the arms and legs. Now the arms can be bent and the doll made to sit or kneel. If the arms are made as long as the legs, the doll can be placed on all fours and turned into an animal!

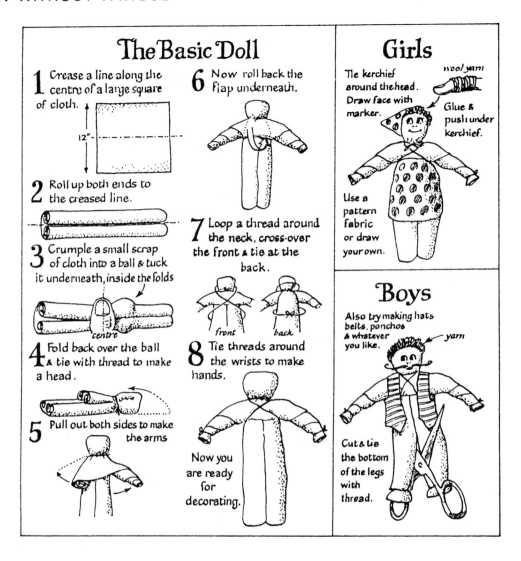

The Basic Doll

1 Crease a line along the centre of a large square of cloth.

12"

2 Roll up both ends to the creased line.

3 Crumple a small scrap of cloth into a ball & tuck it underneath, inside the folds

centre

4 Fold back over the ball & tie with thread to make a head.

5 Pull out both sides to make the arms

6 Now roll back the flap underneath.

7 Loop a thread around the neck, cross-over the front & tie at the back.

front   back

8 Tie threads around the wrists to make hands.

Now you are ready for decorating.

Girls

Tie kerchief around the head. Draw face with marker.

wool yarn

Glue & push under kerchief.

Use a pattern fabric or draw your own.

Boys

Also try making hats belts, ponchos & whatever you like.

yarn

Cut & tie the bottom of the legs with thread.

A Woolly Doll

Very Quick

You may already be familiar with woolly dolls from memories of your own childhood. If so, you will need no help from me! If the idea is new to you, I suggest you make a doll yourself, then show your child how to do it. Your help will probably be needed when it comes to the binding and tying part. Start by making a small hank for the arms by grouping three fingers together and winding the wool over them about ten times. (The thickness of the wool will be the deciding factor.) Carefully slip

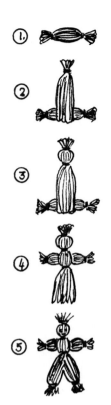

the wool off your fingers. Bind round and tie the hank at both ends to make the wrists as in illustration (1). Lay the hank aside while you make a longer and fatter one to be the rest of the doll. Separate out all the fingers on one hand and wind over them as before. (Wind round about twenty times.) Pick up the arms and poke them into the body hank before you slide it off your fingers. If you don't put the arms in at this stage, the loops of wool that make up the body hank can get out of order, and it is then more difficult to insert the arms. Bind and tie the body hank very near the top (2), the loops will be cut later, to make the hair. A little lower down, bind and tie again to make the face and the neck (3) Slide the arms up tight against the neck. Make sure they are of equal length each side of the body and bind and tie them in place (4). Separate out the rest of the hank to make the legs. Bind and tie round each ankle. Cut the loops of wool on the doll's head to represent a crew cut, and add wool features if you wish. (5)

A Straw Dancing Dolly

Quick

Pam Rigley,
Toy Librarian

This energetic little doll makes a delightful novelty toy. It is soon made from plastic drinking straws and a few beads—all held together with button thread. With the help of gravity, it can be made to dance like a tiny puppet, and its bead feet will tap out a tattoo on the tabletop. It is attractive to many children, but because of its light weight and tiny size it may be particularly suitable for some of the children for whom this book is written.

Materials
- Plastic drinking straws
- A bead for the head, or a cotton ball as shown in the illustration on the next page
- Four smaller beads for the hands and feet
- Button thread

129

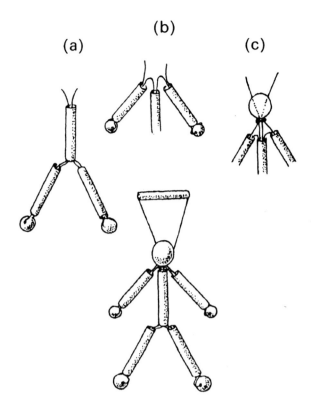

Method

First cut the drinking straws to be the right size to represent the body, arms and legs. Cut a long piece of button thread. Begin at the neck and pass the thread down the body, then down one leg, through a bead (a foot) and back up the leg. Now carry on with the other leg. Pass the thread down it, through the bead for the foot, and back up the leg and the body. Hopefully you now have two threads emerging from the neck end (a). Use one for threading up each arm—down the straw, through the bead and back up the straw (b). Knot the arm threads together, then pass them through the head bead. If you are using a cotton ball, thread them through with a needle (c). Finally, make a dangle handle from a small piece of straw. Finish off by passing one thread through the dangle handle and tying it to the other.

A Pipe Cleaner Doll

Quick

Pam Rigley,
Toy Librarian

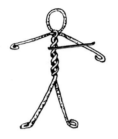

This little doll is made from two pipe cleaners. With a little imagination the basic shape can soon be dressed to make an inhabitant of the dolls' house, or perhaps a tiny 'pocket pal'.

The centre of one pipe cleaner is bent round your finger to make a circle for the head. The ends are bent outwards to form the arms and the tips are folded in to make the hands. The other pipe cleaner is threaded through the head circle, twisted together to make the body, then separated out for the legs. The ends are bent over to form the feet. Roll a piece of paper hankie into a ball and glue it in the head circle to form the face. Alternatively, you can make a fabric face by wrapping a tiny amount of polyester fibre in a circle of double tights material, moulding it to the head and tying it securely at the neck. The body can be padded with a little polyester fibre, and the whole doll will look more glamorous if it is bound in flesh-coloured wool. Add features, and dress as appropriate.

A Doll on a Button

Quick

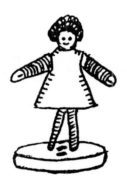

This little doll is a variation on the one above. Originally I made dolls on buttons as people for a road layout. They could stand independently and be moved about easily. To add a little variety to life, I have also used them as counters on a board game.

Materials
- A large coat button with a rim.
- Two pipe cleaners.
- Flesh-coloured wool for binding arms and legs.
- Wool for hair.
- A scrap of old tights material and polyester filling for the face.
- Embroidery or sewing cotton for the features.
- Scraps of fabric for the clothes (felt is ideal).

Method
Hold the button rim downwards. To make the legs and body, take one pipe cleaner and poke it down through one hole in the button and up through another. Make the legs the same length and pull

131

them up firmly so that the centre of the pipe cleaner lies close to the underside of the button. Stand the button on the table and check that it does not wobble. If the rim is not thick enough, the pipe cleaner will protrude and the button will rock about. Find another button with a thicker rim! The finished character must not be top heavy, so keep the legs short. Twist the pipe cleaner about three times in a suitable place to make the body. Leave the ends free for the moment. Take the second pipe cleaner. Hold the ends together. Place your little finger in the centre and twist the pipe cleaner round it—about twice—to make the head and neck. Splay out the ends to make the arms. Attach the body to the head and arms by hooking the body ends over the shoulders—like braces. Twist the surplus round the body. Now to finish the arms. Decide on their length in proportion to the body and bend the surplus pipe cleaner ends back towards the neck. Give each arm a twist or two to make it firmer and to make sure the wire end of the pipe cleaner is safely tucked in. Now the basic skeleton is finished.

Next, some character is needed. Pad out the face with a scrap of polyester fibre. Cover it with a double layer of tights material, tie firmly round the neck and trim away any surplus material. Embroider the features and add some wool hair with long and short stitches or French Knots. To finish off the job, bind the arms and legs with flesh-coloured wool—optional if you are making a character wearing long sleeves and trousers!

A Lavender Doll

Quick

This little brooch doll evolved from some tactile medals I made for a child with multiple disabilities. She was deaf/blind and had only limited movement in one hand. I noticed this was often held near her chest, so (for want of a better inspiration) I made her a collection of little bags that could be safely pinned to her tee shirt within reach of her groping hand. Each bag was covered with a distinctive material like fur fabric. Some also had a noisemaker inserted in them—like a small tin with a pebble inside which

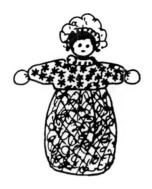

would vibrate and rattle. One was filled with lavender. This caused the little girl to turn her head in order to investigate the lovely smell. Spurred on by this modest success, I made her another lavender bag in the shape of a dolly. The little head was just a ball of polyester fibre covered with tights material. The bodice was just a scrap of cotton print cut T-shaped and sewn up the sides. The lavender was contained in her skirt which was made from fine net. A nappy pin with a safety head was sewn to the back. An unexpected spin off from this simple little doll was that everyone passing by seemed to notice it—and therefore the little girl! I am sure she enjoyed the stroking and attention it brought to her.

A Small Pop-up Dolly

Quick

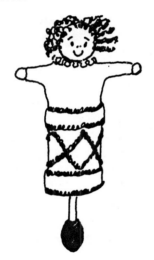

This little toy is small and light. It makes a novelty toy for a gentle child with small hands. It is not suitable for babies, who may be tempted to chew it! It is based on the traditional pop-up doll. The head and dress are attached to an empty plastic film container. A stick attached to the head protrudes through the bottom of the container. Move the stick up and down, and the doll can be made to disappear inside the container and 'pop-up' to surprise everybody!

Materials

- A plastic film container.
- Two wooden beads, one for the end of the stick, the other for the head. The head can also be made from a little ball of polyester fibre covered with material from a pair of tights.
- A short length of thin dowel (say 18 cm, 7″) to fit the holes in the beads. (A sartay stick might do.)
- Thin material for the dress.
- Thicker material to cover the container. Bits and pieces for decoration—wool for hair, pink or brown felt for hands, lace for collar etc.
- Felt pens or sewing cotton for the features.
- PVA adhesive.

Method

Prepare the film container by drilling a hole in the centre of the bottom. Check that the dowel fits in it fairly loosely. Using PVA, stick an uncoloured wooden bead to one end of the dowel, or make a soft head. For this, wrap a small amount of polyester fibre round the head of the dowel. Cover it with a circle of double thickness tights material and squash it into a nice round shape. Gather the edge of the material tightly round the dowel to make the neck. This is a fiddly job. Try to smooth out the creases on the face side of the head. They do not matter at the back where they will be covered by hair or a hat. I find it best to bind the head lightly to the stick while I arrange the creases at the back, then bind it FIRMLY in place and give it a liberal application of adhesive where it folds round the dowel. This is the 'belt and braces' approach, and should make sure the head will never pull off. Check that either the bead head or the soft one will fit easily into the container. There must still be room for the arms and dress.

While the PVA is drying, cut out the dress from thin material. Fold it in half and cut out a shape like a letter T. Make sure that when the sides are sewn up the dress will be wide enough to fit round the top of the container. Put right sides together and stitch up the side seams. Oversew for added strength. Turn right side out. Cut out two tiny felt hands. Turn in the ends of the sleeves, push a hand inside each end and stitch in place. If you have used a bead for the head, cut a hole in the centre of the top of the dress, just large enough to take the dowel. If you have made a soft head, the hole must be a little bigger to make room for the surplus material round the neck. Hold the hem of the dress round the container and have a trial run. If the doll pops up and down as intended, attach the dress firmly to the head—stick and bind, or stick and stitch. Stick and bind the hem of the skirt to the top of the container. Now tidy up the container. Stick on a cover cut from the thicker material. Make the cover a little longer than the container and gather it round the bottom. For extra strength, the cover should also be stitched to the bottom of the dress, where it covers the rim of the container. Finally, add all the embellishments—features, hair, a hat perhaps, and a collar to hide the untidy neckline. (A scrap of lace gathered into a frill is effective!) Finally, add some trimming to the container.

A Sock Dolly

Quick

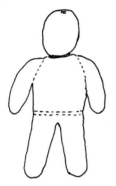

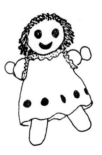

Materials

- An old sock, the longer the better.
- Polyester fibre.
- Scraps of felt and wool for features and hair.
- Scraps of fabric for the clothes.

Method

Cut the foot off the sock and reserve it to make the arms. Think of the rest of the sock in three sections—head, body and legs. Pin where you think the neck and hips will be. Now start with the legs. Lie the sock flat on the table. Cut through both thicknesses of material from the ankle end to just below the pins that mark the hips, and round off the feet. Take out all the pins, turn the sock inside out and stitch up the bottoms of the feet and the inside leg seams. Do this very securely with two rows of stitching and oversew the raw edges, otherwise the sock may fray easily and your seams could pull apart. Turn the sock right side out and stuff the legs with polyester fibre. Stitch across the body, just above the tops of the legs. This keeps the stuffing in place and helps the doll to sit down. Stuff the body and tie (or gather) round the neck. You now have half a doll with legs and a plump little body, but as yet no head or arms. Run a thread round the top of the sock. Unthread the needle, leaving the thread dangling. Add the stuffing to fill the head, gather up the thread, rethread the needle and again fasten off very firmly. Cut two arms from the reserved sock foot and round off the hands. Sew two sausage-shaped arms—strong seams as before. Stuff them and stitch them to the body securely. Sew on felt features or embroider them, and add wool hair. Cover the head with large French knots for a curly hairstyle. For a straight cut, wind wool over some thin card and machine or hand stitch down the middle to keep the strands of wool in order. Cut the wool where it bends over the card. Tear the card away from the stitching. Sew the wool hair to the doll, arranging the stitching along the line of the parting. Make some simple dolls' clothes and play can begin.

The undressed sitting down doll illustrated was made by a nine-year-old. She used a long green sock. The heel made the doll's sit-upon and the legs were made from part of the foot. She used the rest of the foot to make the arms, and folded down the top of the leg to make a cosy hat.

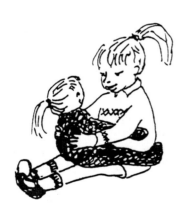

A Life-sized Baby Doll

Long-lasting

Fran Whittle and her team,
All Saints Arts
and
Youth Centre, Sussex

Fran's dolls make life-sized companions and can be dressed in proper clothes complete with zips, buttons, bows and poppers.

Materials
- A Babygro, outgrown perhaps or from a jumble or car boot sale.
- Stretch fabric for the head. Fran recommends cotton stockinette.
- Polyester fibre with the CE safety mark on the bag.
- Wool, felt and thread for hair and features.

Method
First stuff the Babygro. Then make the head. Cut a strip of stretch fabric appropriate to the size of the Babygro. A young baby's body is approximately $3\frac{1}{2}$ times the length of its head, and its neck is very short. Stitch the short sides of the fabric together to make a ring of material. Run a thread along one edge, gather up and fasten off securely. This is the top of the head. Turn the fabric right side out. Run another thread around the open (neck) end. Unthread the needle and leave the thread dangling. Stuff the head, rethread the needle, draw up the

running thread and again fasten off securely. Put the head on top of the Babygro and join them together with several rounds of stitching. The doll will have a floppy head, just like a real baby. This makes it very appealing.

To make the face, first cut the features out of felt. Start with the eyes. These should be positioned half way down the face (or lower) and fairly wide apart. Pin them in place. Do the same with the mouth (and nose?). Try moving the pieces about a little to see how the expression changes. When you are satisfied, stitch the pieces in place and remove the pins. The hair can be made of wool as for the sock dolly on p. 135. (I know of one dolly who was crowned with a cap of brown fur fabric. Very fetching!) Select some suitable clothes from the 'cast offs' and your doll is ready for some tender loving care.

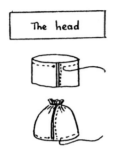

The head

See also
A Weather Doll, p. 112.

PUPPETS

Puppets come in all shapes and sizes and hold a fascination for children and adults alike. A furry glove puppet cleverly manipulated by an adult is certain to attract the attention of a small child, and everyone laughs at the witty dialogue between a ventriloquist and his dummy. The word 'puppet' seems to cover anything from an instant hand-held rod puppet such as a cat's head made from a paper bag stuffed with newspaper, to an elaborate stringed puppet with magnificent clothes and a prominent part in a professional play. The ones included here are all meant to be used by children, and can probably be made by them too.

Card-Plus-Finger Puppets

These simple little puppets come to life when the child's finger is poked through a hole in the cardboard. Here is the simplest of all.

A Worm Puppet

Very Quick

Cut out a rough circle of card, large enough to cover the child's fist, and colour it brown (to represent the earth). Make a hole in the centre. The child pokes a finger through this and a wiggly worm appears! It might be the character in the following jingle:

There's a worm at the bottom of my garden,
And his name is Wiggly Woo.
There's a worm at the bottom of my garden,
Oh dear! What shall I do?
He wiggles all night, and he wiggles all day,
The people all turn round and say,
'There's a worm at the bottom of my garden,
And his name is Wiggly Woo!'

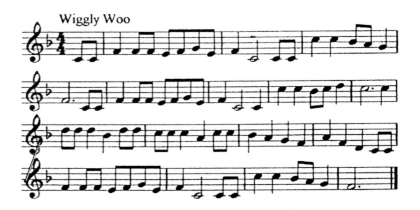

Wiggly Woo

An Elephant Puppet

Very Quick

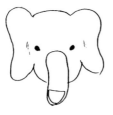

This time draw the head of an elephant, and cut a hole at the top of his trunk. The child's finger poking through this can make the elephant appear to be searching for food, trumpeting, or lumbering along with his trunk swinging from side-to-side.

Nosy Rosie

Quick

Make a Nosy Rosie puppet from a polystyrene drinking cup. This idea comes from an American book *1-2-3 Puppets* by Jean Warren. Jean cuts a hole in the side of the cup for a finger to poke through (Nosy Rosie's nose), adds features with

138

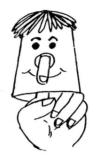

felt pens and glues on a few wisps of wool to represent hair. Then Nosy Rosie can roam round the room sniffing at whatever takes her fancy. This little ditty is sung to the tune of 'Here we go round the mulberry bush'.

Here comes old Nosy Rosie,
Nosy Rosie, Nosy Rosie,
Here comes old Nosy Rosie
Sniff sniff sniffing flowers (or what you will).

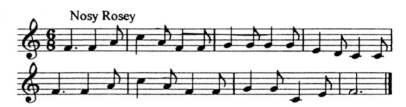

Clothes-peg puppets

Turn a spring clothes-peg sideways on and pinch the end. Immediately the clothes-peg appears to be opening its mouth! The simple little puppets that follow make use of this movement. Basically, they are just circles of card glued, or attached with Blu-tac to a wooden peg. Three examples are described, but once you have the idea, no end of characters can be created ... all capable of talking to each other in profile.

A Fish

Quick

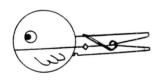

Begin with a circle of thin card, say 6cm (2¼″) in diameter. If you make it larger, it may be too heavy to stick to the average clothes-peg. Colour the fish. Cut it in two, making the bottom jaw smaller than the upper. Attach both pieces to the peg, just in front of the spring. Use a strong glue e.g. U-Hu or Evostick and hold the pieces in place until the glue sets. (Blu-tac will also do the job.)

A Duck

Quick

This is based on the same circular shape, but has a bill added to the circle before cutting it out. It comes in handy as a Mother Duck for the rhyme about the

139

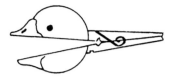

five little ducks on p. 143, who went swimming one day, and it is also useful for 'Old MacDonald had a Farm'. Other animal heads can be made on the same principle.

An Alligator

Quick

Another variation on the theme, but this time the jaws are lengthened, and they are separated by a zigzag cut to represent the fierce teeth.

Finger puppets

Finger puppets are excellent for sparking off imaginative play and, of course, they make splendid small presents. Any Mum, Auntie or Grandmother who makes a few to keep by for an emergency will bless the day she had such forethought. They are great for long journeys, as a little reward, or as a consolation in a crisis.

Now for some hints on how to make this satisfactory little toy:

Instant

To make a finger puppet in a jiffy, simply draw a face on a finger, yours or a child's, and wrap a handkerchief or tissue round it. It is immediately clothed in a hood and cloak! Keep this rudimentary clothing in place with a rubber band.

Very Quick

If you have an old pair of fabric gloves in something like a flesh colour, cut off the best fingers and embellish them as you fancy or as play dictates. Put your finger inside the potential puppet. This makes it easier to work on. Draw the eyes and mouth with felt pens. If these do not show up well, indicate the features with a few stitches. Stick on some wool hair (PVA adhesive). Add some felt clothes—stitched or stuck—or use layers of lampshade fringing for a 1920s dress!

Finger Puppets to Knit

Quick and easy

One of the highlights of the play sessions at our toy library at Kingston-upon-Thames is Music Time. The children and their Mums and Dads gather in a semicircle round the piano to join in the action songs and finger plays. It is noticeable that the ones which include finger puppets hold the children's attention best. Their hand movements are larger and freer and even the shy ones will join in. When the ritual of giving out the puppets begins, the chosen child carries round the bag. Some children take the nearest ones, others pick out their favourite colours. It is obvious from the delight on their faces that they consider the best part of the session is about to begin! The puppets have an educational value too. We can discuss the colours, count them, help each other put them on and, if there is an argument, negotiate a swap. We ring the changes between 'Two Little Dicky Birds', 'Two Grand Ladies' and 'Five Little Ducks Went Swimming One Day'. Of course, these are not the only examples of nursery rhymes that can be acted out with finger puppets.

The Basic Pattern

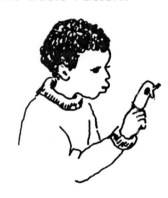

This takes a proficient knitter about 20 minutes to knit. I have 'outworkers' among some very senior citizens and children who are just learning to knit. They welcome this useful little knitting job, which can be completed before they grow tired or bored. The demand for the 'Two Little Dicky Birds' is constant, and I am grateful for their help.

Materials
- Knitting needles—say 10 or $3\frac{1}{4}$.
- Wool—DK or four ply. (If thinner perhaps use double.) Bright, light colours, no navy blue!

Method
Cast on 14 st.
K2 (or 4) rows garter st. (Plain knitting)
K about 24 rows stocking st, (1 row plain, 1 row purl). Use a little common sense here. Imagine the finished finger puppet and the size of the finger of the child in question. Use fewer stitches or knit less rows if necessary.
Break off the wool and thread it through the stitches. Draw up the stitches and stitch up the back seam. (Your puppet now looks like a fingerstall.)

Stuff the head with a small ball of Polyester fibre—or similar.
Bind round the neck with matching wool.

Two Little Dicky Birds
Knit the basic pattern twice. Use a different colour for each bird. Make the eyes in black wool (French knots) and add a felt beak, diamond shaped. Stitch it in place with cotton. In case you have forgotten the rhyme, here it is:

> (Put a finger puppet on each index finger)
> *Two little dicky birds sitting on a wall,*
> *One named Peter*
> (hold one puppet up high)
> *One named Paul*
> (hold up the other)
> *Fly away Peter*
> (hide him behind your back)
> *Fly away Paul*
> (hide him too)
> *Come back Peter*
> (bring him out from behind your back)
> *Come back Paul*
> (bring him out too)

At the toy library we usually finish off the rhyme by letting the dicky birds greet each other—because they are so pleased to meet up again!

Two Grand Ladies
Knit the basic pattern above, but after about twelve rows of stocking stitch change to a flesh-coloured wool for the face. Finish off as before. Now make the ladies as grand as possible. Use odd scraps of felt and fabric trimmings, and let your imagination get to work. Perhaps one lady might have an elaborate wool hair-do with a flower on top, while the other wears a felt hat with a feather in it. Embellish a silk dress with sequins or decorate a

velvet one with lace. Good taste doesn't come into it—the more exotic the better!

This is the rhyme:

Two Grand Ladies met in the lane
  (Have them on your index fingers, hold them
    apart and gradually bring them together.)
Bowed most politely, bowed once again
  (Make your fingers match the words and bow to
    each other)
'How do you do?'
  (One finger bows)
'How do you do?'
  (The other bows)
And 'How do you do?' again.
  (Both bow)

Five Little Ducks

For the little ducks, knit the basic pattern five times in yellow. Add black French knot eyes and orange felt beaks. For the Mother Duck, either represent her bill by the fingers and thumb on your hand working in opposition and opening and shutting on each 'quack', or she can be more enduring and spectacular made as a snapper puppet, p. 146.

Here is the rhyme:

Five little ducks went swimming one day,
Over the pond and far away.
  (Wear the ducks on one hand and make them
    'swim' across the pond.)
Mother Duck said 'Quack, quack, quack',
  (Use your other hand or the snapper puppet in
    time to the words.)
And FOUR little ducks came swimming back.
  (Bend one finger down)

Four little ducks went swimming one day, ... etc.

Repeat with one less duck each time until ...
And NO little ducks came swimming back.

Last verse . . .
Mother Duck went swimming one day,
Over the pond and far away.
Mother Duck said 'Quack, quack, quack',
And FIVE little ducks came swimming back.

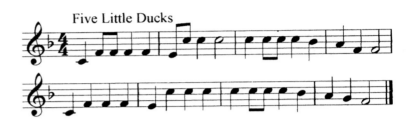

Five Little Ducks

A Snowman
Knit the basic pattern in white, add a black felt hat, features and a brightly coloured scarf.

A Guardsman
Start in black for his trousers, change to red for his tunic. Give him a flesh-coloured face and add a few extra rows to top him with a black busby. Make his brass buttons with yellow French knots and finish him off with a felt belt.

Finger puppets with arms

Quick

These little people are slightly more complicated to knit than the ones above, but look more realistic and can be used for story telling or holding conversations.

Materials
- Knitting needles and scraps of wool including flesh colour, as for the finger puppets above.

Method
The front and back are identical. They are knitted separately, then partly stitched together so that the hands can be added.

Here is the pattern. Knit it twice.

Cast on 8 st.
K2 rows plain, 12 rows stocking stitch.

144

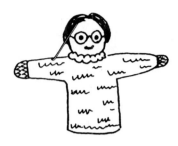

The Arms
Cast on 4 st. K into the backs of the first 5 st., then K to the end of the row.
Cast on 4 st. P into the backs of the first 5 st, then P to the end of the row. (16 st.)
K 1 row.
P 1 row.
Cast off 6 st. to make one shoulder, K to the end of the row.
Cast off 6 st. For the other shoulder, P to the end of the row. (4 st.)

The Head
Break off the body colour, leaving a tail, which will come in useful later for sewing up the top of the sleeve. Tie in the flesh colour for the face.
K into the front and back of the first stitch, K 2, K into the front and back of the last stitch.
P 1 row.
Increase 1 st. at the beginning and end of the next row (8 st.)
P 1 row.
Work 4 rows stocking stitch.
K 2 together at both ends of the next row, (6 st.)
P 1 row.
K 2 tog. at both ends of the next row. Break off wool and thread it through the remaining 4 st. (Do not cut it off. It will be needed later to sew up one side of the head.)

Knit the other half of the puppet the same way.

Finishing off
With right sides together, join the front to the back from the top of the head and along the top of the arms. Now add . . .

The Hands
Using flesh colour, pick up 9 sts across the end of one sleeve. K 4 rows stocking stitch. Break off the wool and thread it through the stitches. Sew up the side of the hand. Repeat the process at the end of the other sleeve. Complete the joining up, under the arms and at the sides.

145

Turn the puppet right side out. Stuff the head with a scrap of polyester fibre or similar and tie round the neck. Bring your puppet to life by adding features, wool hair and, perhaps, some adornments like a sequin brooch, French knot buttons, a lace collar or a fetching hat.

The body of the standard puppet lends itself to variations. It can be knitted in two colours to represent Jeans and a jersey, fabric clothes can be added ... even 'props' like a tiny duster can be stitched to one hand on a pom-pom ball tucked under a child puppet's arm. To make a baby, simply reduce the pattern by casting on less stitches—say 6—and working fewer rows.

MORE SIMPLE PUPPETS

Mother Duck Snapper Puppet

Long-lasting

Mary Hurst

The snapper puppet is made from three squares of plastic canvas, but the face and bottom jaw squares are extended to make the bill (*see* diagram). When the three pieces are assembled, the back of the head acts as a spring, keeping the bill closed. Pinch the cheeks at the appropriate moment and the puppet opens its mouth to say 'Quack' on cue!—all due to the remarkable properties of plastic canvas!

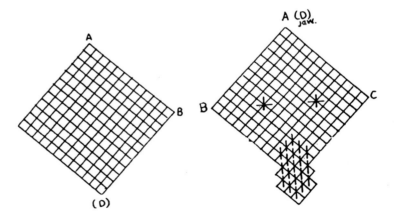

Back of head   Face and bottom jaw

Materials
- Seven-mesh plastic canvas (from a craft shop). This has eight bars, seven holes, to the inch.
- Wool—tapestry or DK, perhaps used double. White for the head, yellow for the bill. Black for the eyes.
- A tapestry needle. This has a large eye and a blunt point.

Method

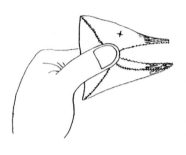

Cut out a square of canvas for the back of the head. Make it 13 bars each way (12 holes). Before cutting out the face and bottom jaw as in the diagram, I find it helpful to run a tacking stitch from point A, through the middle of the bill to its tip. It is important that the tip of the bill lines up with point A. It is easy to snip off an extra bar by mistake and make the bill lop-sided.

Now for the stitching. Cover the back of the head first, using cross or tapestry stitch. Next, cover the face, making the bill yellow and adding the eyes. These *must* be stitched in at this stage, as it is impossible to add them once the puppet is assembled. Then stitch the bottom jaw in the same way, but omitting the eyes, of course! Finally, join all the appropriate edges ... AB on the face to AB on the back piece, and AC to AC. Make extra stitches at A to make sure the point is covered. Oversew the bottom jaw to the back by joining DB to DB and DC to DC. In yellow, oversew all round the edges of the duck's bill.

Now squeeze her cheeks to make her open her bill and appear to 'Quack'.

Glove puppets

Bought glove puppets may be too large and heavy for small hands, but it is easy for anyone handy with a needle to make one just the right size. First cut out a paper pattern. Place the child's hand on a piece of paper with the fingers and thumb in the position they will adopt when working the puppet. Most children like to use their thumb for one arm, their index finger for the neck and their middle finger for the other arm. The ring and little fingers are tucked into the palm. A few children prefer to use two fingers to work the head and two for the arm not filled with the thumb. Draw round the child's hand in his chosen position, making a very generous seam allowance. Cut out the puppet in double material and tack round the seams. Try it for size before stitching properly, then decorate according to character. A slit up the back of the puppet's dress can make it easier for some children to put their fingers in the right place.

If you have no particular character in mind, you might like to make a percussion player. For this all you need to do is make a glove puppet and stitch metal buttons to his hands. Now he can play the cymbals in time to music on the radio!

A Vilene Puppet

Quick

Cut out a hand puppet, as described above, in heavy duty Vilene and stitch round the edge. The child can decorate the Vilene with felt pens and create any character she wants. Before the colouring begins, it is wise to slip a piece of paper inside the puppet in case a felt pen used on the front bleeds through to the back.

A Glove Puppet made from a Sock

Instant or Quick

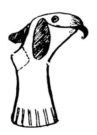

Some readers may remember the TV puppeteer Sharri Lewis and her endearing glove puppet 'Lamb Chop'. This type of puppet is very easy to make and in its simplest form is definitely instant! Just put your hand into the sock and part of the way down the foot. Tuck in the toe between your fingers and thumb to make a mouth. Now you can move your fingers and thumb apart and together again to make the sock appear to be talking. In this crude state the puppet will probably soon lose its 'mouth'! To prevent this, withdraw your hand and make a few stitches at the sides of the mouth to keep the pocket (formed by the tucked in toe) folded in.

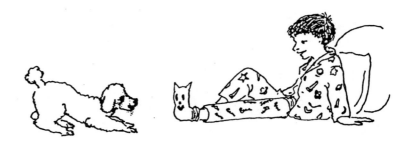

Use felt to add floppy ears and a tongue. Black button eyes can look effective. With wool, sew eyebrows, nostrils and perhaps whiskers. I like to use a sock with a long leg that will cover part of my arm. For small children choose a child's sock of the appropriate size.

Long-lasting toys

TWO TOYS FOR YOUNG CHILDREN

This chapter describes some slightly more complicated toys that I have devised for individual children. My prowess with the sewing machine or with woodworking tools is not advanced. Anyone with basic skills and a love of 'making things' might like to read on. I have described the toys and the reasons for making them, but have not always included detailed instructions. These toys have been added as a possible source of inspiration! If you are searching for a special toy to make for a birthday or other celebration, perhaps you will find something below that may start you thinking.

Small, Very Light Bricks

Long-lasting

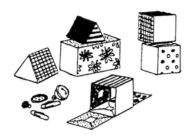

These little bricks are easy to make by hand, but time consuming. The first set was made for a little boy of about two, (let's call him Rupert) who suffered from Epidermolysis Bullosa (blistering skin). The fragile nature of his skin made it essential for him to have lightweight toys that were hygienic. These bricks can go in the washing machine and wash beautifully at a low temperature. Because of their light weight, and novelty value, they can be attractive to other children at the building stage. For satisfactory play, you really need to make quite a few—say at least a dozen.

The bricks are made from squares of plastic cut from margarine or ice cream tubs. Each square is covered with fabric, patchwork fashion, and six are assembled into a cube. Rupert was interested in toys that made a noise, so his bricks had either a few foil milk bottle tops, small buttons, paper clips, or a bell inserted. He could use them for stacking and building in the normal way, or they could become a sound discrimination game. He could shake and rattle them, and group together all those he considered to have the same contents.

Materials

- Plenty of plastic tubs and boxes. If the plastic is thin and pliable, use it double. There will be a lot of wastage, because only the flat areas are useful.

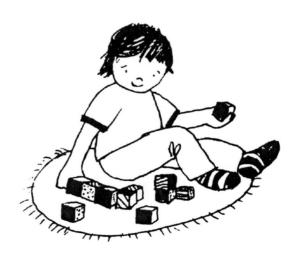

- Scraps of material. Cotton is best.
- Stiff card or thin ply for a template, size at your discretion. 5 cm square (2″) is suggested. This is too large to be swallowed, but is a convenient size for small hands.
- Noisemakers if you want your bricks to rattle. Avoid pasta, rice etc., as these will not wash!

Method

To make one brick

Use the template and cut six squares from the flat parts of the plastic containers. Lay one square onto the material. Draw round it, then cut out the fabric square, allowing at least 1 cm seam allowance all round. Fold the top and bottom seam allowance over the plastic and lace the edges together with a long zigzag tacking stitch. Turn in the other two sides and also zigzag them together, making the corners as neat as possible. Repeat for the other five squares. Hold two squares, right sides together, and oversew both fabric edges together. Make a few extra stitches at the corners for added strength. Open them out, and add two more squares, making a strip of four. Add the two remaining squares, one each side of the strip, to make a cross. Fold it up to make a cube. Oversew all the unstitched sides. If your brick is intended to rattle, remember to insert the noisemaker before you close the last seam! Make as many more bricks as you need.

Note

It is possible to make these bricks in a variety of shapes, and so extend their play value, e.g. cut two squares, 5 × 5 cm (2 × 2″) and four rectangles 5 × 10 cm (2 × 4″) and you have a double-sized brick. For a ridged roof, cut three squares (or rectangles) and two equilateral triangles, sides 5 cm. For a pyramid, cut one square and four triangles. I have also made sets of 'stacking and nesting' cubes by this method. I omitted the sixth side of every cube and made each one slightly larger (or smaller!) than the previous one, so that finally all would fit inside the largest.

The Peg Bus

Long-lasting

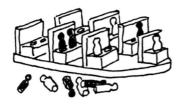

This simple wooden toy was originally made to my requirements, in a sheltered workshop. The prototype was made for a child of seven with Cerebral Palsy. He was able to put large plastic peg men into the holes in the toys designed for them and his therapist felt he was ready for a more challenging activity—like putting smaller pegs in smaller holes! For this toy, 'dolly' clothes pegs were ideal, and gave their name to the toy. The split part (which would normally clip the washing to the line) was sawn off, leaving a neat little peg man ready for painting. The Peg Bus turned out to be a very successful toy and gave pleasure (and useful training) to many children who needed to practise their hand-eye co-ordination.

The bus was roughly the shape of a flat iron and measured about 30 cm (12″) from end to end. It was meant to represent a minibus, with the driver in front and the passengers sitting in pairs behind him. The wood block seats had holes drilled in them. These were slightly larger than the pegs, and quite deep so that the passengers would fit in them securely. A small piece of plywood was glued to the back of each seat. This helped the child to direct the pegs into the holes. The pegs were coloured in pairs so that the toy could also be used for colour matching—the two yellow ones sharing the same seat. (The driver wears a white coat!) The bus was not fitted with wheels. This not only simplified the construction, but also prevented the bus from moving just as the child was aiming a peg at a hole.

Once the child had loaded all the passengers, the Peg Bus could be used for story telling. It might go on an outing. On the way, the passengers could chat to each other, perhaps tell jokes, quarrel or even be sick! (Always a popular diversion!) Once the destination was reached, the passengers needed to be unloaded, perhaps arranged in a circle to enjoy a 'pretend' picnic and then, of course, loaded onto the bus again for the return journey. Plenty of peg handling for the child in question!

Note
These truncated dolly pegs can have many more uses. They are excellent for home-made pattern-making peg boards. Simply drill rows of holes in some sturdy ply or MDF and provide a quantity of coloured pegmen.

For children who cannot manage to play board games such as Ludo, Snakes and Ladders, etc. the normal way with small counters, it may be worth while to make the baseboard in wood, drill holes as appropriate and substitute pegmen for counters.

RAG BOOKS

Rag books are usually associated with babies and toddlers, but the ones described below have been specially made for older children. Rag books are virtually indestructible and, therefore, well worth making for children in hospital or respite care, for they can be used over and over again. They can be dribbled on, even chewed, and are soon restored to their first glory by a swirl in the washing machine.

Note
If you think your book will need frequent washing, avoid using felt. This useful non-fray material will shrink and the colours often run. Use a woven material instead.

How to Make a Rag Book

1. Use plain material for the pages. Unbleached calico is ideal. It is cheap, very strong and easy to work with.
2. Decide on the size of your proposed book, then cut the plain material into rectangles *twice* the size of each page. Each rectangle will be doubled over, so that the fold in the fabric makes the turning edge of the page.

3. Open out the fabric to single thickness ready for you to start work. A simple and effective way to make a picture book is to use the design on children's nursery prints. These may illustrate nursery rhymes, space men, animals, etc., or follow the trend of the moment with pictures of TV favourites. Cut out the pictures you want and tack them to the pages of the book. Stitch round the edges with a very short machine stitch and cover this with a narrow, close zigzag stitch. If you would like to add words or a story to the pictures, a laundry marker pen will do the job.

I like to decorate my pages collage fashion, using fabrics with interesting textures and colours. Sometimes a picture may have a door or windows to open, so that the child can peep into the house, or perhaps a leaf will lift up, revealing a tiny insect underneath! All very time consuming, but fun to do, and much appreciated by the recipient of the book. You may be efficient in the use of fabric markers and, instead of sewing, wish to draw your own pictures.

4. When a double page is finished, fold it so that the decorated sides are together. Machine stitch across the top and bottom of the doubled-over pages, leaving open the side opposite the folded edge. Your work now looks like a bag lying on its side. Turn the page the right side out. Make sure you poke out the corners. Now your book is under way. Make as many more pages as you think necessary.

5. When all the pages of the book are finished, make two more fabric bags to be the covers— only the top one needs to be decorated. I make mine very slightly larger than the pages and stiffen them with a fabric stiffener, such as heavy-duty iron-on Vilene or pelmet stiffener.

6. Finally, assemble the book. Tack two pages together (four thicknesses of material—add another page if you think your machine will not protest) and machine down the open edges. Then hold the pairs together and

oversew by hand through all the thicknesses of fabric to make the spine of the book. Do not pull the thread too tightly or the pages will not lie flat. The result is probably a strong, but untidy mess! Bind this with a strip of contrasting fabric, turning in the ends and hemming it in place along the length of the spine. Oversew or ladder stitch across the ends to stop them unfolding.

Note
Here is a tip which may be helpful to children who have difficulty in turning over a page. Try making each one a slightly different size so that the edge of one overlaps the next. I made a successful book for a child with Cerebral Palsy using this system. In this case, the pages were also stiffened like the cover. This prevented them from rucking up as the child tried to turn them.

A Versatile Picture Book

Long-lasting

Every factory-made rag book is designed for babies, so it is impossible to find one for an older child with learning difficulties or hand function problems, who might really appreciate such a toy. Open this Versatile Picture Book and you might think you were looking at a photograph album with each snap neatly framed and protected with a plastic cover. Examine it more closely, and you would find that one side of each frame is not stitched to the page. Whoever owns the book is at liberty to take out a picture and slot in another as the mood dictates. Perhaps the present topic is the school trip. When this is no longer hot news, the photos could be exchanged to feature the family and pets or whatever! This Versatile Picture Book is unique, because it has easily turned pages, is indestructible, washable (at a low temperature) and can be made interesting for a child of any age—just like the family photograph album. I have made several of these books for children with very special needs. One was for a girl of eleven, who could not walk without support and was unable to speak. She was also partially sighted. My aim was to try to widen the scope of her unsupervised playtime by adding the rag book to her toy box and offering her an alternative to shaking various noisemakers or banging two toys together. Because of her poor sight, her book needed to be on a larger scale. Windows of $20 \times 20\,cm$ $(8 \times 8'')$ seemed suitable. A window was stitched to the pages on the right hand side of the book only. This could make it easier for her to focus on them and to learn to turn the pages over. I drew large, clear pictures of her toys, clothes, family car and familiar items around the house. These could be used in rotation. I added some black pages decorated with diffraction stickers bought off the roll at the local toyshop. When the sun shone, these showed up brilliantly and gave her particular pleasure.

Another special rag book was made for Rupert . (You may remember his 'Small Light Bricks', p. 152) His book contained ten pages and—as illustrated— there was a window on each side. These were the right size to hold a photo or a picture postcard. His first illustrations were of people he knew and places he had visited.

Here is the shopping list for making a Picture Window Rag Book.

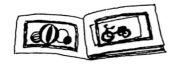

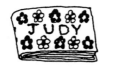

Materials
- Fabric for the pages. Unbleached calico is ideal.
- Clear plastic for the windows. I use PVC from the soft furnishing department of a large store. The plastic must be pliable. It has to accept machine stitching and be able to bend when the pages are turned inside out.
- Black tape or black bias binding for the frames.
- Plenty of pictures. Collect several sets the same size, so that they can be interchanged as required.

Method
Cut out the calico pages twice the width you want and crease down the fold. This will become the leading edge of the page. Next make the windows.

Cut the number you want from the clear plastic. Allow for the frames and make them slightly larger than the pictures you will use. Apply black tape or bias binding to the four sides of the plastic. Now attach the windows to the pages. Take one window and pin it in position. (If the plastic is fairly stiff you may need to tack it.) Machine stitch round *three* sides, leaving unstitched the side that faces the spine. Putting the open side here makes it more difficult for the pictures to fall out accidentally. Stitch another window to the opposite page. Now place the windows face-to-face and stitch across the top and bottom of the page to make a bag, as with the rag book. Turn the bag right side out and you have completed the first page. Make as many more pages as you want, and finish off the book as described above.

A Counting Book for Yasmeen

Long-lasting

Yasmeen was a very intelligent three-year-old. Sadly she had an illness that restricted the use of her arms and confined her to her special chair. She needed table-top toys that were small, light and intellectually challenging. Her counting book was made on the same principle as the rag books above but, bearing in mind Yasmeen's special needs, the pages were considerably smaller (actual size 10 × 14 cm, 4 × 6″). When the book was open a flap could be unfolded from the bottom edges of the front and back covers. These flaps stored the numbers 1–5 and 6–10. Each number was embroidered on a small felt disc backed by a furry Velcro Spot-on. The matching rough half of the Spot-on was attached to a flap. Each page of the book was decorated with items to count. In play, the required number was lifted from a flap and transferred to another rough Velcro spot on the page. The flaps tucked in when the book was not in use and the pages were kept closed with a small button and loop—like a hasp on a precious volume!

Note
To make the book as described you need twenty rough Velcro spots and ten furry ones. It took

many evenings to make the book, but I think the time was well spent. The result was an unusual and special present for a 'frail' child. This is one of those toys where the creator has as much fun as the recipient!

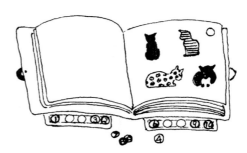

Here—just to start you thinking—are the ideas I used for the pages.

- *One felt house*—with embroidered window boxes and roses round the door. A face looked out of a window and a cat was asleep on the step.
- *Two fish with black sequin eyes*, cut from glamorous gold and silver lycra, and appliquéd to the page.
- *Three little faces*, made in stockinette and slightly padded from the back to give them shape. (Trepunto quilting.) Their hair was made of wool—French knots for curls—and their features embroidered. (Yasmeen's Mother reported that she held little conversations with them.)
- *Four trees in a copse*, cut from fabric with interesting textures. A few embroidered flowers grew in the grass beneath them to add a little extra interest and colour.
- *Five sequin flowers* sparkled in a felt bowl.
- *Six tiny buttons* decorated a felt coat.
- *Seven gaudy felt balloons* were tied together in a tidy bunch.
- *Eight ribbon roses* (bought from a haberdashery stall in the market) grew on a leafy rose bush.
- *Nine sequin stars* twinkled in a dark blue felt sky.

- *Ten small wooden beads* hung on a necklace round the neck of another (larger) face.

The book held one more surprise. Inside the back cover was another cloth flap on which were embroidered two hands with the fingers and thumbs spread out. Yasmeen could open out the flap, match her own hands to the stitched ones, and count her fingers and thumbs.

A Look-and-Listen Book

This book was made for the small children at the toy library. It came out as a special treat on important occasions like birthdays. It also proved to be an excellent way of breaking the ice with a new little member. Because it was not washable, it was a treasured object to be shared between child and adult, and not to be played with unsupervised on the floor! A musical button (from the Craft Depot, p. 184) was positioned on each page, i.e. it was covered in net and the net was then stitched to the page. When pressed, the sound button played a nursery rhyme. This was illustrated on the page.

The book was made in unbleached calico on the same lines as the rag book above, but it was considerably bigger, measuring about 30 cm (12") square. The cover was titled LOOK AND LISTEN in large felt letters, and the spine covered with red and white spotted cotton fabric. Each page was stiffened with pelmet stiffening.

Page one was my first effort. The tune was 'Jingle Bells', so I covered the sound button with net, stitched it to the centre of the page and surrounded it with circles of brightly-coloured fabric, each with a small bell attached by a buttonhole stalk to the centre. As the tune played, the child could run his hands over the little bells to set them jingling.

Page two illustrated 'Twinkle, Twinkle Little Star'. This one was easy! I covered the page with navy blue felt and decorated it with star sequins of different sizes and colours.

Page three was 'Old Macdonald had a Farm', and again this was fairly easy to illustrate. I had several scraps of nursery fabric with farm animals on, so all I needed to do was cut them out, arrange them suitably and appliqué them to the page.

Page four was rather more complicated. The tune was 'The Teddy Bears' Picnic'. Again, I was able to find various teddy bears on nursery fabric. These played in the woods (hiding in the trees, playing a game of ball, etc) and sat round the tablecloth spread out on the grass. I tried to introduce as many different textures into the collage as possible.

The tune for the final page five was of 'Brahms Lullaby' so, of course, it showed a baby asleep in a cot with the moon looking in through the window.

Decorating the pages took a long time, but the finished result gave great pleasure to all its users. The book was kept in a special bag, so remained clean and fresh until (after many months) the buttons eventually became so faint that the tune was barely recognisable. Even then, the book lived on as a picture book, with an adult leading the singing of the nursery rhymes.

Note

Do not remove the little feet under the sound button in an effort to make it lie flatter to the page. If you do, the sound will be muffled.

A TOY FOR OLDER CHILDREN

The Turntable Toy

Long-lasting

You may remember the Revolving Play Table (p. 10) in the chapter on 'Making Play Possible'. This toy is based on that principle. The first one was made for a child with brittle bones. Because of her small size and need to play mainly sitting in her special chair, she was unable to reach further than about 20 cm (8″) and, of course, this restricted her activities. By using a 40 cm (16″) turntable her reach was doubled.

I made a series of heads to fit on the turntable.

A Town Layout

This was based on a circle of MDF. To make the terrain more interesting, I sanded down a thin block of wood until it looked like a low hill, and glued it near to the centre of the circle. A roadway ran round the edge of the layout and across the centre, with a couple of cul-de-sacs added—to give more possibilities for imaginative play. Excluding the roads, the layout was peppered with small holes. These were for holding the many model houses, trees, and other buildings—like the school, Church, hospital etc., and for the street furniture like the phone and pillar boxes. All these were cut from MDF, painted, and varnished. A hole was drilled in the base of each, and a tiny peg inserted. Now the little house, or whatever, could be placed on the turntable head and with the little peg in one of the holes, there it would stay until the child decided to move it. In the original version, I used a piece of matchstick. This was fine for careful children, but could be easily snapped off by the heavy-handed. I discovered some plastic rods, of matchstick diameter, in a shop for model makers. Cut into small pieces, these were ideal for the purpose. Adding a variety of vehicles put the finishing touch to the layout. These were also cut from scraps of MDF. They had no pegs, for they were intended to be pushed around the roads. There were cars of many colours and makes, an ambulance, a fire-engine, a double-decker bus, a coach, a minibus, a removal van, a Police car and an ice cream van, surely enough for any community!

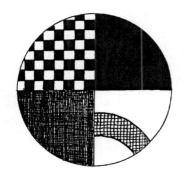

An Open Plan Dolls' House

This had three rooms and a garden. The walls slotted together. The furniture was made from plastic canvas (as used for the Mother Duck Snapper Puppet p. 146) and stitched appropriately. It was strong and washable. The illustration on the next page shows the bedroom. The drawers in the little chest can be removed. Through the door there is a glimpse of the kitchen with its tiled floor and electric cooker. It also has a fridge—with a door that opens—a table and chairs, a tiny bucket made from a plastic lid and a miniature mop made from a tooth pick with a woollen mop head. The far room is the sitting

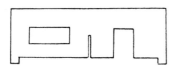

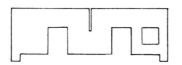

163

room with a comfortable sofa and armchairs complete with cushions and its 'Persian' carpet on the floor. There is also a bookcase with tiny books and of course a TV! To the right is the garden with a lawn and patio tubs filled with bright flowers—planted in Polyfilla in toothpaste lids! The finishing touches are the inhabitants—pipe cleaner dolls (p. 131) and the little plastic wheelchair from a set of Playpeople. This can be pushed from room to room. By revolving the turntable, all the rooms are easily brought within reach of the child.

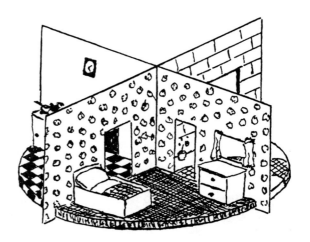

A Farm
This time the top of the turntable was covered with calico and, according to the seasons, fields made from various textured material could be attached to it with Velcro. Brown corduroy represented a ploughed field, pale green terry towelling made passable Spring wheat—and so on. The farmhouse and buildings were made from a plastic canvas but, in this book of home-made toys, I regret to report that the animals and farm implements came from a toy shop!

Presents for children to make

PRESENTS FOR YOUNG FRIENDS

Everyone likes to receive a present. When my own children were small, it was sometimes quite difficult to think of a suitable gift for them to make for a friend or a grandparent. These days the TV Children's Programmes can be a source of inspiration, but in case you miss them here are a few very simple ideas which came in handy in our house as a festival or birthday approached.

Look in the section 'More Quick and Easy Toys to Make', p. 115 and in the section on 'What to do with . . .' (p.178)

PRESENTS FOR ADULTS

Bookmarks

Quick

These can be a suitable present for anyone, whatever their age or sex. They can be produced in a jiffy by the very young, or made with elaborate care by a perfectionist! Here are some suggestions.

A book worm
Draw a curvaceous worm on card. Use this for a template. Place the template on some felt and draw round it. Cut just inside the line—so the pencil mark will not show. Stick on two goggle eyes from a craft shop (or draw them with felt pen, but this is not easy on felt as the outline tends to blur.)

Some ideas for a more conventional bookmark
- Start with a strip of thin card. Decorate it with a freehand design using felt pens.
- Make a pattern using cut and gummed paper shapes from a stationers or toy shop.
- Stick print it, *see* p. 175.
- Decorate it with pressed flowers or leaves. Fix each item to the card with small dots of PVA adhesive, and protect the surface with clear sticky-backed plastic.
- For children who are learning to embroider, stitch a book mark in stranded cotton on a strip of suitable fabric and back it with ribbon.

Fridge Magnets

Quick

Materials
- Small round magnets, sold for the purpose in craft shops. They can be attached to any small flat surface. Make sure you have the magnet the right way up or it could repel the fridge door instead of sticking to it!
- A strong adhesive like Evostick or Araldite (a job for an adult!)
- A surface to decorate. Choose from the suggestions below.
    1. *Cut out a fairly sturdy card shape.* Decorate it with felt pens. Cover the surface and edges

with clear sticky-backed plastic. Attach a magnet.

2. *Use a small metal or plastic lid from a jam jar*. Cut out a circle of thick paper or thin card to fit inside the lid. Decorate it with a picture or design, and stick it to the underside of the lid. Glue a magnet to the top.

3. *Fill the underside of a lid with Polyfilla*. Poke in melon seeds, dried peas, chick peas etc., or sea shells if you live near the sea. The creator of this one needs to have nimble fingers and be a quick worker. The pattern must be finished before the Polyfilla sets.

4. *Mix up a small amount of Playdough* (p. 175). Roll out a small piece to be the base. Cut it to the shape required. Decorate it—perhaps with an initial formed from a sausage of Playdough? Leave it to dry out or bake it in a very low oven. Paint it. (Use the paint as thick as possible or the Playdough may go soggy.) When dry, protect it with a couple of coats of Polyurethane varnish. Attach the magnet to the back.

5. *Do more elaborate modelling using Fimo* (p. 77).

Lavender Bags

Quick

These make very acceptable gifts for elderly friends and—if the smell of lavender is relished—are enjoyable to make. I like to sit a small group of children round a table and place a pile of lavender on a large sheet of newspaper between them. First they must strip the lavender from the stalks and put it into cereal bowls. The empty stalks are neatly stacked to one side as the job progresses. When all the lavender is stripped, the newspaper and stalks are cleared away, and the making of the lavender bags can begin. For young children, the simplest way is to spoon a pile of lavender from the cereal bowl into the centre of a circle of thin fabric. This might be voile, fine net curtain, muslin etc., and about the size of a saucer. Then they must gather up the fabric and tie a ribbon round the lavender. This is usually a job for an adult. Some older

167

children can do it for themselves if they first make a row of running stitches round the circle where the ribbon will go. Then, making sure the needle is safely stuck in a pin cushion—they can fill the inside of the circle with lavender, draw up the running stitches and fasten off the cotton. Now the lavender is safely encased, and it is an easy job to tie the ribbon bow.

See also
A Lavender Doll, p. 132.

A Pomander

Quick, but allow time for it to dry out

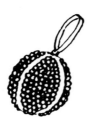

Choose a well-shaped orange. Mark it vertically into four equal segments with narrow strips of Sellotape. This shows where the ribbon will go and defines the areas to be filled with cloves. Using a fine knitting needle or a cocktail stick, make a hole in the orange just deep enough to take the stalk of a clove. Push one in, then make another hole, and so on until every section is filled. Do not squeeze the orange or the juice may dribble out. Roll the pommander in ground cinnamon and gently wrap it in foil—or waxy paper from the inside of the cereal packet. Keep it in a warm cupboard for about six weeks, while it dries out and shrinks. Finally, remove the Sellotape and tie up the orange with pretty ribbon.

See also
Pebble Painting—p. 79.

Odds and ends

This chapter contains all the bits and pieces that I have found hard to include elsewhere. In it you will find more detailed help for several of the crafts and hobbies mentioned in the Alphabet (pp. 75–83) and recipes for making your own play materials—like finger paint and playdough.

PAPIER MÂCHÉ

In this book, papier mâché is mentioned in the section on Crafts and Hobbies, p. 79. Perhaps the use of papier mâché in toy making is a technique new to you. If that is so, and you would like to try it, read on for some hints, which should help you to achieve really good results.

First, here are some general thoughts on the versatility of the technique. It seems strange that a material as floppy as a sheet of newspaper can, with the help of flour and water paste and a little patience, be laminated to make a substance as strong as wood—*and* the cost is minimal!

It can be used to make dishes and pots, and it can also be used as a modelling medium. For this, the newspaper is torn into small pieces and soaked in a bucket of water until it is truly saturated. Then it is squeezed as dry as possible and mixed with stiff flour and water paste. This makes a grey and soggy mess! It is easy to convert this into sausages, potatoes, bananas, apples, etc. When painted (and protected with polyurethane varnish), these are ideal for 'shop' play. This mixture can also be used to model faces for glove puppets or make a hundred and one other 3D items, like haystacks and hedges for a farm layout or a tunnel for the model railway.

The paper

- Always use unglazed paper. It breaks down better and absorbs the paste well. Before you begin, collect some ordinary newspaper with words on it, and some with coloured printing—perhaps the pictures and advertisements in the paper. Using black and white and coloured paper in alternate layers makes it easy to apply them evenly. It is obvious which parts have been covered, so 'holidays' and weak spots can be avoided.

- Mass produced paper has a 'grain' and will easily tear into a strip if you tear with the grain. Sometimes this runs horizontally across the page, sometimes vertically. Trial and error will show the direction on the paper you use. Tear from top to bottom, and then from side to side. One way you will get a neat, straight tear, the other way the tear will be unpredictable.

- Always tear the paper. This gives a ragged edge and helps each strip to blend with the next. If you cut the paper, you will get a hard edge to each piece and this makes for a less smooth finish.

- The paper should be well pasted, but not too soggy or it will take ages to dry out. Make sure all edges are well stuck down and there are no bubbles, or the surface will be uneven and the article will not be strong.

- The final layer should be applied in cheap white unglazed paper—the unprinted edges of the newspaper might do. Alternatively, the finished (and thoroughly dry) article can be given a coat of white matt paint before being decorated.

- It is essential to be patient over the drying out stage. Apply the paint too quickly and the result will be patchy and disappointing.

- Finally, protect the toy or object with at least two coats of polyurethane varnish. This will make it spongeable and helps to protect the corners from scuffing.

Mixing the Paste

- 1 heaped tablespoon of plain flour.
- A little cold water—enough to mix the flour to a smooth paste.

- About 400 ml of boiling water.
- A Pyrex jug.

Put the flour in the jug. Add the cold water very gradually, squashing out all the lumps, until the mixture looks like thick cream. Stir continuously, and gradually pour in the boiling water until you have made a pint of paste (500 ml). For safety's sake, it is best for one person to hold the jug and stir, while another person pours in the boiling water. This is NOT a job for children.

As you add the boiling water, the flour will partly cook. The mixture becomes thicker and more translucent. Once it has cooled, it is ready for use.

Note
It has a limited 'shelf life', but will store in the fridge for a few days.

Using papier mâché as a modelling medium

This can be a messy job (beloved by children!), so first protect the child and his surroundings. Then together, tear up some newspaper into small pieces and put them all in a bucket. Soak for as long as possible, (say overnight), then squeeze nearly dry and add a little flour and water paste or PVA adhesive. Mix well. The resulting grey sticky mess is now ready to be moulded into vegetables for a shop, a tunnel for the model railway—or what you will. It is advisable to make the object fairly small at first, let it dry out overnight and then add some more grey sticky mess, gradually building up the shape you require. A large soggy item made in one go may lose its shape and droop, and will certainly take ages to dry out.

Dishes and Pots

If you fancy a less messy way of using papier mâché try this:

For a small dish, tear the paper into strips or small pieces. Cover the back of a saucer with cling film and apply the scraps of newsprint evenly all over it using cold water paste or PVA adhesive (diluted a little for economy!). Add the next layer in coloured newsprint. When sufficient layers have been built up—say five or six—leave the dish to dry out overnight. When the papier mâché dish is hard and quite dry, it can be removed from the saucer and the cling film peeled away. If the edge is not very even, it can be trimmed with a pair of old scissors. If the layers of paper look as if they are separating out, it is worth while sticking small pieces of newspaper over the edge, all the way round. This will make a neater and stronger job, but will mean postponing the painting until the paste has dried. First the newsprint must be covered with a layer of white paper, or a coat of white paint. Emulsion paint is ideal for older children who can work tidily and not spill it! Powder paint or poster paint will do almost as well, but will tend to flake off if applied too thickly. If the child has the patience, suggest several thin coats rather than one thick one. When this undercoat is dry, the design can be applied. The finished dish will benefit from a coat (or two) of polyurethane varnish to protect the surface and make it spongeable.

To make a pot, perhaps use a plastic flowerpot as a mould, turn it upside down, cover it with cling film and then build up the layers of paper as before.

Note
If you are not a woodworker and would like to make really strong, large toys, it is possible to do so using cardboard from cartons combined with newspaper and paste. Further information can be had from Intermediate Technology Publications Ltd, 103–105, Southampton Row, London, WC1B 3HH. Tel: 0207 436 9761. Recommended Book, *Appropriate Paper-Based Technology* (APT) A Manual, Bevill Packer.

PRINTING

Printing is mentioned in the alphabet of crafts and hobbies p. 80. The little girl illustrated there is having a wonderful time preparing to print with her hands. This is a much enjoyed, messy activity which has even more play value if the resulting prints can be put to some use. One obvious end-product is to print some wrapping paper and, maybe, a card to go with it.

Handprints

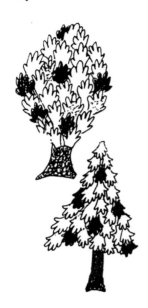

Handprints can be cut out and, if you have sufficient, might be added to a large bird shape to represent the feathers, or they can be arranged as deciduous trees with the fingers pointing upwards, or point them downwards and you have a fair representation of a coniferous tree!

Mount a single hand print on thin card, turn it this way and that to see what it reminds you of, add a lolly stick handle and you might have a simple fish stick puppet. Add a few more fingers and you have an octopus! These simple hand prints so beloved by toddlers can lead on to more exotic designs.

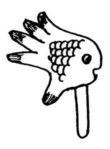 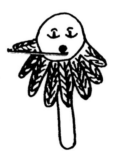

A paint pad on a saucer is less messy than a tray full of paint and is more suitable for printing smaller shapes. Mix powder paint fairly stiffly, then place a pad made from a few layers of felt on a saucer. Impregnate the pad with the paint. Make sure it does not dry out by adding a little more paint when needed.

Thumb and Finger Prints

Start with a thumb print for a body, put a finger print above it for a head, draw ears, a tail and whiskers and you have made a convincing back view of a cat!

174

Another old favourite is a baby chick. Use a yellow thumb print for the body, add a fingerprint for the head and finish off by drawing in the eye, beak and legs. After a few experiments, I guess the printer will improve on this, and think up his own ideas.

Printing with Objects

A carrot cut in half will make excellent spots that can represent balloons on a sheet of wrapping paper. Potatoes of a suitable shape can be sliced in half to make the basis for a Humpty Dumpty and they can be carved (probably by an adult) to give a raised shape, say the child's initial.

Stick Printing

This gives scope for even more originality and invention. The end of a pencil or ruler, a cotton reel or the side of a wooden clothes-peg can all be pressed into the paint pad in the saucer and the colour and shape transferred to the paper.

String Printing

Find a wooden block—or some thick cardboard cut to shape. (Make it into a block by laminating several shapes together.) Draw a curving line over the top surface of the block. Make sure the line does not cross over itself. Cover the line with a trail of water-resistant glue (e.g. U-Hu). Press fairly thick string onto the glue. Make sure it sticks securely. Trim the ends and wait for the glue to dry. Press the block onto the paint pad and print large sheets of all-over patterns. These are useful as wrapping paper or book covers, etc.

Small printing blocks for more delicate work are on sale in many general craft shops.

PLAYDOUGH

Four Recipes

There are several ways of making playdough. Which one you choose may well depend on the contents of your store cupboard! If mixed thoroughly, all the recipes will make a pliable dough which will set really hard. Wrapped in a plastic bag or stored in a screw-topped container, the dough will keep in the fridge for about a week. On damp days, the salt in the dough may tend to make it sticky. Just add a little more flour. If the playdough cracks and does not hold together, it is too dry. Add a few drops of water and mix them in well. Do not use playdough with a child who has cuts or broken skin on his hands—the salt in the dough will make the sore places sting.

Recipe One
(The easiest)

- 1 cup plain flour
- $\frac{1}{2}$ cup salt
- A little water

Mix the dry ingredients together and add the water very gradually until you get a dough that looks like pastry.

Recipe Two
- 2 cups plain flour
- 1 cup salt
- 1 cup water, perhaps with food colouring or powder paint added to it
- 2 tablespoons cooking oil

Put all the ingredients in a bowl and mix together thoroughly.

Recipe Three
- 3 cups plain flour
- $1\frac{1}{2}$ cups cooking salt
- 3 teacups water
- 6 teaspoons cream of tartar
- 1 dessertspoon cooking oil

Put everything in a saucepan and mix it all together. Stir it over a low heat until it binds together and comes away from the sides of the pan. Leave it to cool.

Recipe Four
- $\frac{1}{2}$ cup cornflour
- 1 cup salt
- $\frac{1}{2}$ cup water

Blend everything together in a saucepan. Cook over a low heat until the mixture thickens, stirring all the time to avoid lumps. Leave to cool.

BUBBLE MIXTURE

Here is the recipe:

- 1 pint of water—or $\frac{1}{2}$ a litre
- 2 tablespoons concentrated washing-up liquid (or a little more if it is normal strength)
- 1 tablespoon glycerine (from the chemist). This is essential for strong bubbles, but add too much and the mixture becomes sticky.

Store in a plastic squash bottle.

FINGER PAINT

Two Recipes

Recipe One
- Flour or cornflour. About a cupful should be sufficient for use with one child.
- A little powder paint.
- Water to mix.

Put the flour and paint in a bowl and mix them together. Gradually add the water, squashing out all the lumps, until the mixture is like thick cream. If made with cornflour, this mixture, placed on a Formica-topped table or baking tray has a strange amoeba-like quality. It can easily be made to change its shape. Push it into a pinnacle, and it will subside into a pancake. Push against the edge, and it will bulge out somewhere else. Children find this fascinating!

177

Recipe Two
- About a cup of soapflakes (*not* detergent)
- A little powder paint
- A little water

Mix as for Recipe One and beat it into a smooth paste. Water it down a little so that it is easy to spread. I am told this recipe can be used to paint patterns or pictures on the side of the bath, but I haven't tried it myself!

WHAT TO DO WITH ...

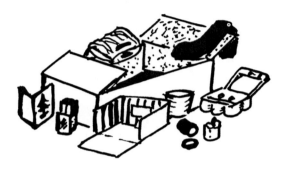

A Cardboard Box

This is perhaps the most versatile scrap material of them all. If presented with a large cardboard box, most children will instantly put their imagination to work and convert it into (in their eyes) a truly splendid toy.

- It can become a house, a car, boat, bus or train or even a hidey hole.
- It makes a splendid counter for a shop.
- Turned upside down, it can become the shell of a tortoise, the child underneath, crawling along with it on his back.
- With a square hole cut in one side, it is transformed into a TV set with the child inside, ready to present the programme.

When our children were about four and six they saw, outside the electrical shop, a pile of cardboard boxes put out for the dustman. A quick word with the shopkeeper, and these were soon stacked one inside the other and brought home in triumph. All was ominously quiet in our son's bedroom, and I went to investigate. The floor was covered with an intricate maze of cardboard boxes, their flaps raised to cover the gaps. The children were somewhere inside, happily crawling through this astounding construction! This is one use of the cardboard box which would never have occurred to me!

See also
A Play Table for Bed or Floor, p. 9.
A Play Corner, p. 9.
A Play Box, p. 10.

A Shoe Box

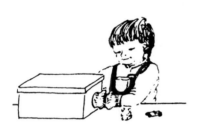

- This can make an instant bed for a doll or teddy. A folded tea towel will do for a mattress, with two man-sized tissues for sheets and a third one folded to make a pillow. Rectangles of fabric cut with pinking shears will pass for blankets. Collect several boxes and all the dolls and animals can go to hospital!
- Cut a hole in one end. Secretly put a tactile object in the box. Hold the lid on firmly and invite the child to put his hand into the box and guess what is inside.
- Cut one (or two) holes in the lid, and you have an instant first posting box, ready to receive cotton reels or square bricks.
- Stand the box on end. Keep the lid in place with rubber bands and cut a slot near the top to represent a letterbox. Now it is ready to swallow a pack of playing card 'letters' each one posted individually!
- Cut down two corners so that the long side will fold outwards and form an extension to the bottom. This can become a room for a dolls' house. Now the walls can be decorated with home-designed wallpaper, the floor and its extension carpeted with fabric, windows cut out and hung with curtains. Pictorial stamps make excellent pictures for the walls, kitchen foil will pass for a mirror and the lid from a toothpaste

tube will make a bucket or a container for a pot plant. Dolls can be cut from old magazines etc, or made as Instant Dolls, p. 127, or Pipe Cleaner Dolls, p. 131. Furniture is easy to make from matchboxes, thin card and Sellotape, or whatever comes to hand. (When you were a child did you ever make little chairs from conkers, with pins for legs and more pins for the backs, with wool woven between them?)

At the end of playtime, the floor extension can be folded up, the lid replaced, and the quickly-made toys inside will be safely stored until next time.

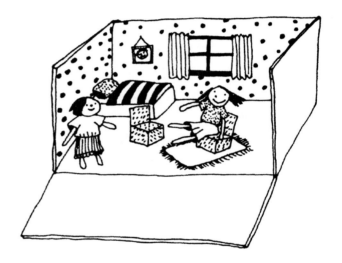

An Egg Box

An empty egg box is enough to intrigue a toddler for a considerable time—just flapping the lid, opening and closing it, feeling in all the little recesses. It can also be used ...

- for sorting large buttons.
- as a cash till for shop play.
- as a stacking toy. Cut out the recesses and turn them upside down. Let the children decorate them with felt pens, then pile them one on top of the other.

- as a Humpty Dumpty. Join two segments together with masking tape, and decorate to represent Humpty Dumpty. Sit him on the side of an egg box (painted red to represent the wall) and he can fall off when the punch line of the rhyme is reached.
- As a colour matching game. For this you need two egg trays. Turn them upside down so that the recesses become mounds. Felt pens to the fore and colour a mound on one tray. Copy it on the other. Continue like this until all the mounds on one tray have a matching mound on the other. It may be necessary to repeat some colours. Leave one tray intact, but cut out all the mounds on the other. These can now be placed over the correct colours on the whole tray.
- In Korea the teachers of young children make a delightful game using an egg box, a pair of stamp tweezers (large and with blunt ends) and little cotton balls (from a craft shop) in six bright colours. The children pick up the balls, one by one, with the tweezers and must put all those of the same colour into the same recess.

An Odd Sock

- Collect a few small ones and half fill them with fish grit. Rice or dried peas are lighter, but will not wash. Sew across the top of the sock and use as beanbags, or as a stacking toy—especially useful for children who find it difficult to grasp and release.
- Use longer ones as Instant feely bags. Simply put in a spoon, or an egg cup, or a marble, or a crunchy paper bag from a packet of crisps, or a few large buttons—take your pick from whatever suitable that comes to hand—and tie a knot in the leg.

See also

A Manx Feely Cushion, p. 44.
A Sock Dolly, p. 135.
A Glove Puppet made from a sock, p. 148.

A Yoghurt Pot

- Collect several and use them as a lightweight stacking and nesting toy. To make them look more elegant, cover the sides with stamp-sized scraps of coloured paper glued on with PVA adhesive.
- Use three for an Instant 'Find It' game. (You may know this as the three card trick.) Your child watches you hide a small object under one pot. He sees you change the positions of the pots then tries to guess which one hides the object. He lifts the pot to check if he is right. Take turns to hide the object and, when it is your turn to guess, sometimes get it wrong!
- Use several pots for a target game. The children must try to throw (or flick—as in Tiddly Winks) small objects into them. The yoghurt pots may need stabilising. A pebble in each may do the trick, or make loops of masking tape and stick them to the table, or use blobs of Blu-tack.

See also
A Special Bubble Blower, p. 102.
A Cup and Ball, p. 122.

Matchboxes

- Use them to make dolls' house furniture. Place some together to make chunky arm chairs, a chest of drawers, a dressing table, or use two covers joined together with one tray to make a grandfather clock! The trays used singly will make a baby's bed, a fireplace or, lined with baking foil, even the kitchen sink!
- Stuff a matchbox with a tissue and cover the outside with paper or Fablon, and you have a *Quick* lightweight brick. Make lots more.

See also
Matchbox Puzzles, p. 49.
A Pop-up Matchbox, p. 121.

Note
Make sure the abrasive strip on the side of the box is always covered.

A Plastic Film Carton

- Put in a bell or some small buttons (etc.), glue on the lid and sew the carton into a fitted fabric cover—or crochet one—so that there is no chance the child can remove the lid, and you have another noisemaker to add to the collection.
- Use in sand and water play. The cartons with recessed lids make excellent rollers for the sandpit and will soon mark out a roadway to fit a small car. For water play, punch holes in the sides to make a mini-sprinkler.
- Put one outside the dolls' house as a dustbin.

See also
Some Small Light Rattles, p. 31.
A Sound-matching Game, p. 32.
A Small Pop-up Dolly, p. 133.

A Plastic Carrier Bag

- Turn one upside down. Cut out a head hole in the top (once the bottom) and two armholes at appropriate place at the sides, and you have an Instant cover-up for messy play.
- Cut round one in a spiral to make a long plastic strip about 5 cm (2″) wide. Use this to knit or crochet a bag (large needles or hook). This makes a useful, and quick-drying container for the bath and water play toys. (You may need several carrier bags. The lettering and pattern on the plastic will make an attractive design as it is worked into the bag.)
- Use, pinned to the sheet, as a rubbish bag for a child in bed.

Old Christmas Cards

- Use for conversation and for sorting. Together pick out all the ones with animals, or children—or snowmen, etc.
- Cut out the pictures carefully and remount them to make new cards, or notelets or labels for presents.

- Combine them with other pictures or a child-painted background, to make collage pictures.

See also
    Christmas Card Jigsaws, p. 49.
    Mary Digby's Special Scrapbook, p. 52.
    Making a Scrapbook with a Theme, p. 52.
    Playing Alone Lifesavers, p. 83.

USEFUL ADDRESSES

Organisations

Action for Leisure
c/o Warwickshire College, Moreton Morell,
Warwickshire, CN35 0BL
Tel: 01926 650 195;
Web-sites: www.sed.kel.ac.uk/special/
schools.html; www.eparent.com;
www.etoys.com.
A resource centre with a wide selection of
toys, games and equipment. Items to
purchase. Data base of information,
reference library of books and videos etc.

*National Association of Toy and Leisure
Libraries*
68, Churchway, London, NW1 1LT
Tel: 0207 387 9592; Fax: 0207 383 2714;
e-mail: admin@natll.ukf.net;
Web site: www.charitynet.org/-NATLL.
For information about your nearest toy
library, a useful book 'Switch into Action'
etc.

Educational suppliers

Hope Education
Orb Mill, Huddersfield Road,
Oldham Lancashire, OL4 2ST
Tel: 0161 633 6611;
e-mail: orders@hope-education.co.uk;
enquiries@hope-education.co.uk;
Web-site: www.hope-education.co.uk.

NES Arnold
Novara House, Excelsior Road, Ashby Park,
Ashby de la Zouche, Leicestershire,
LE65 1NG
Tel: 1871 6000 192; Fax: 0800 320 0001;
e-mail: orders@nesarnold.co.uk;
Web-site: www.nesarnold.co.uk.

Craft suppliers

Craft Depot
Somerton Business Park, Somerton, Somerset,
TA 11 6SB
Tel: 01458 27 47 27; Fax: 01458 27 29 32;
e-mail: craftdepot@aol.com;
Web-site: www.craftdepot.co.uk.

Toys etc.

Brookite
Brightly Mill, Oakhampton, Devon, EX20 1RR
Tel: 01837 53315; Fax: 01837 53223;
e-mail: info@brookite.com;
Web-site: www.brookite.com.
For kites of all sizes, and the materials to make them if you wish. Also 'Wind Things' – spinners, twisters, wind wheels to look spectacular in the garden. Unfortunately they do not deal with individual mail-orders. Write for a catalogue and look for them in the shops!

Dowling Magnets
Lee Valley Technopark, Ashley Road,
London, N17 9NL
Tel. Mail-Order Express: 08700 12 9090;
Fax: 020 880 4136;
e-mail: sales@dowlingmagnets.co.uk.
For magnets of all descriptions, and lovely magnetic toys.

The Great Little Trading Company –
Practical products for parents and kids
1 Broad Plain, St. Philips, Bristol, BS2 0ZZ
Tel: 08702 41 40 81; Fax: 08702 414083;
Web-site: www.gltc.co.uk.

Hawkin's Bazaar
Hawkin and Co., St. Margaret, Harleston,
Norfolk, IP20 0HN
Tel: 01986 782536; Fax: 01986 782468;
e-mail: sales@hawkin.co.uk;
Web-site: www.hawkin.co.uk
A good source of small novelty toys.

James Galt and Co. Ltd
Brookfield Road, Cheadle, Chesire, SK8 2PN
Tel: 0181 428 9111; Fax: 0181 428 6597;
e-mail: mail@galt.co.uk;
Web-site: www.galt.co.uk.
For toys and craft kits. Mostly retail, but there is a department that deals with individual orders.

Living and Learning
5–7, Pembroke Avenue, Waterbeach,
Cambridge, CB5 9QP
Tel: 01223 864894; Fax: 01223 864464;
e-mail: lfraser@tribune.com.
For science kits, unusual games and puzzles.

Mail Order Express
39, Sherrard Street, Melton Mobray,
Leicestershire, LE13 1XH
Tel: 08700 129 090;
e-mail: averilchester@arbon-watts.demon.co.uk
For a wide selection of toys by post.

Spiel and Holz Design
Available by mail-order from:
Myriad, The Buckman Building,
43 Southampton Road, Ringwood, BH24
Tel./Fax: 01425 402000;
Web-site: www.myriad,purplenet.co.uk.
For beautiful and unusual wooden and fabric toys.

Printed in the United States
73875LV00003B/111